STUDY GUIDE TO
GERIATRIC PSYCHIATRY

A Companion to
The American Psychiatric Publishing
Textbook of Geriatric Psychiatry,
Third Edition

STUDY GUIDE TO
GERIATRIC PSYCHIATRY

A Companion to
The American Psychiatric Publishing
Textbook of Geriatric Psychiatry,
Third Edition

Lloyd Benjamin, M.D.

Clinical Professor, Department of Psychiatry and Behavioral Sciences
University of California–Davis School of Medicine
Sacramento, California

James A. Bourgeois, O.D., M.D.

Associate Professor of Clinical Psychiatry and Allan Stoudemire
Professor of Psychosomatic Medicine, Department of Psychiatry and Behavioral Sciences
Director, Consultation-Liaison Service
University of California–Davis School of Medicine
Sacramento, California

Narriman C. Shahrokh

Chief Administrative Officer, Department of Psychiatry and Behavioral Sciences
University of California–Davis School of Medicine
Sacramento, California

Dan G. Blazer, M.D., Ph.D.

J. P. Gibbons Professor of Psychiatry
Department of Psychiatry and Behavioral Sciences
Duke University Medical Center
Durham, North Carolina

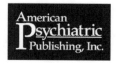

American Psychiatric Publishing, Inc.

Washington, DC
London, England

Manufactured in the United States of America on acid-free paper
10 09 08 07 06   5   4   3   2   1

ISBN   1-58562-263-X
ISBN-13   978-1-58562-263-4

First Edition

Typeset in Revival BT and Adobe's The Mix

American Psychiatric Publishing, Inc.
1000 Wilson Boulevard
Arlington, VA 22209-3901
www.appi.org

Contents

Questions

Answer Guide

Page numbers in the Answer Guide refer to *The American Psychiatric Publishing Textbook of Geriatric Psychiatry*, Third Edition.

Visit **www.appi.org** for more information about this textbook.

| | | |

Purchase the online version of this Study Guide at

www.cme.psychiatryonline.org

and receive instant scoring and CME credits.

Chapter 1

The Myth, History, and Science of Aging

Select the single best response for each question.

1.1 Hayflick is noted as having determined that

    A. Cells continue to divide at a fairly even rate throughout life.

    B. Cells double at a rate inversely proportional to age.

    C. Frozen cells thawed years later now divide at a rejuvenated rate; memory of the number of prior doublings is "forgotten."

    D. Death of a cell line is usually due to faulty laboratory techniques.

    E. The only human cells that may be immortal are mixoploid cells, such as HeLa cells.

1.2 Aging is usually considered

    A. Necessarily confined to the latter years of life.

    B. To result in a decline in efficiency of function, reduce homeostasis, and terminate in death.

    C. To not particularly involve changes in striated musculature.

    D. To result in diminished capacity for storage of drugs.

    E. To result in declines of tyrosine hydroxylase, cholinesterase, and monoamine oxidase.

1.3 Major advantages of aging include all of the following *except*

    A. The aged are much better citizens and interested in public issues and political affairs.

    B. Older workers are stable but have more absenteeism.

    C. In general, older persons are much less likely to be the victims of crime than people of other age groups.

    D. Older persons maintain voluntary participation in community organizations, churches, and recreational groups.

    E. Social Security and other pension systems have improved the economic status of older persons.

1.4 Timing of age-related change is thought to involve all of the following *except*

    A. Cell loss within clusters of the hypothalamus.

    B. Telomere shortening and cellular senescence.

    C. Oxygen free radicals.

    D. Decrease in the immune competence and alterations in the regulation of the immune system.

    E. Loss of glycated forms of human collagen in tendon and skin with age.

1.5   The differential in life expectancy between men and women is thought to involve all of the following *except*

    A. Death rates by accidents and other violent causes are higher for men than for women.
    B. Ischemic heart disease is consistently higher for men than for women.
    C. There is greater incidence of cigarette smoking among men.
    D. Malignancies are less frequent among males than among females over most of the life span.
    E. There are differences in smoking habits between men and women.

Chapter 2

Demography and Epidemiology of Psychiatric Disorders in Late Life

Select the single best response for each question.

2.1 The "old-old" populace (older than age 85) is projected to reach what number of persons by the year 2050?

A. 10 million.
B. 12 million.
C. 20 million.
D. 25 million.
E. 27 million.

2.2 The geriatric population is expected to increase to how many by the year 2030?

A. 30 million.
B. 40 million.
C. 50 million.
D. 60 million.
E. 70 million.

2.3 Case identification in geriatrics is particularly germane because

A. Distinction between a case and a noncase is easily established.
B. Epidemiologists cannot assist the clinician in identifying meaningful clusters of symptoms.
C. Many of the symptoms and signs of a psychiatric disorder in late life may be ubiquitous with the aging process.
D. Clinicians particularly favor case identification based on severity of functional impediment.
E. Most older adults ideally fit the psychiatric diagnosis they receive.

2.4 The NIMH ECA program (1984) established the two most prevalent disorders of the elderly as

A. Depressive and anxiety disorders.
B. Depressive and cognitive disorders.
C. Depressive and psychotic disorders.
D. Anxiety and cognitive disorders.
E. Anxiety and psychotic disorders.

2.5   The most frequently reported psychiatric symptom(s) of the elderly is (are)

   A. Depression.
   B. Fatigue.
   C. Problems with sleep.
   D. Anxiety related.
   E. C and D.

2.6   Suicide in the elderly

   A. Is highest in the 65–74 sector.
   B. Is highest in the 78–84 sector.
   C. Is inversely correlated with age.
   D. Is most pronounced in white men older than 70.
   E. Has demonstrated a cohort effect of an increased rate with more modern manufacture of domestic gas.

2.7   Major depression has *not* been associated with

   A. Having functional limitation.
   B. External locus of control.
   C. Poorer self-perceived health.
   D. Perceived loneliness.
   E. Being unmarried.

Chapter 3

Physiological and Clinical Considerations of Geriatric Patient Care

Select the single best response for each question.

3.1   Falls in the elderly

    A. Are frequently multifactorial.
    B. Involve one-third of all community-dwelling elderly every year.
    C. Predict considerable morbidity.
    D. Promote risk for decline in instrumental activities of daily living.
    E. All of the above.

3.2   Urinary incontinence in the elderly is

    A. Most frequently stress incontinence in men.
    B. Most frequently overflow incontinence.
    C. Most frequently urge incontinence.
    D. Seen in up to one-half of community-residing elderly.
    E. None of the above.

3.3   The musculoskeletal system is affected in which of the following ways?

    A. Decrease in skeletal muscle mass.
    B. Increase in number of type II fibers.
    C. Age-associated changes in muscle mass and strength may be modified by exercise.
    D. A and B.
    E. A and C.

3.4   Considerations in geriatric prescription should include all of the following *except*

    A. Volume of distribution.
    B. Absorption.
    C. Renal clearance.
    D. Oxidative metabolism in the cytochrome P450 system.
    E. Change in elimination half-life.

3.5 All of the following are true of the aging nervous system *except*

A. Significant neuronal loss occurs in the locus coeruleus.
B. Aging neuronal synapses may be decreased in the substantia nigra.
C. Aging neuronal synapse size may be decreased in the substantia nigra.
D. Aging neuronal synapse size may be increased.
E. Protein and myelin content of the brain decreases.

3.6 Which of the following is true of cognition in normal aging?

A. Crystallized intelligence changes with age.
B. Fluid intelligence begins to improve in the middle of the sixth decade and thereafter.
C. Practical intelligence may be stable or even improve with age.
D. Aging adults do not lose the ability to sustain attention over long periods.
E. Short-term memory is affected.

3.7 Ocular changes include which of the following?

A. Weakening of the ciliary muscle.
B. Photooxidation leading to yellowing of the lens.
C. Decline in ability to view objects at rest.
D. A and B.
E. A, B, and C.

3.8 Vascular changes of the elderly consist of all of the following *except*

A. Elevated sympathetic nervous activity with increased level of circulating norepinephrine.
B. Cardiac and vascular surface cell receptors less sensitive to norepinephrine.
C. Beta-adrenergic response of the heart during exercise is exaggerated.
D. A lower maximum heart rate.
E. Less cardiac emptying.

3.9 Gastrointestinal system changes of the elderly include

A. Fewer myenteric ganglion cells.
B. Diminished acid and pepsin production by the stomach.
C. Diminished function of liver, gallbladder, and pancreas.
D. Diminished ability of liver to manufacture binding proteins.
E. Diminished liver transaminases and alkaline phosphatase.

3.10 Hormone levels are affected in all of the following ways *except*

A. Decrease in growth hormone.
B. Decrease in dehydroepiandrosterone.
C. Decrease in cortisol.
D. Increase in parathyroid hormone levels.
E. Increase in sex-hormone binding globulin levels.

Chapter 4

Neuroanatomy, Neurophysiology, and Neuropathology of Aging

Select the single best response for each question.

4.1   The limbic system

   A. Is involved in complex behaviors including the elaboration and expression of emotion.
   B. Is involved in learning and memory.
   C. Does not include the amygdala.
   D. A and B.
   E. A and C.

4.2   EEG recordings of normal aging would not be expected to show

   A. Small increase in beta frequency.
   B. Small increase in theta frequency.
   C. Small increase in alpha frequency.
   D. No significant increase in delta frequency.
   E. Dominance of frequencies in the alpha range.

4.3   EEG changes with dementia include

   A. Decrease in delta and theta activity.
   B. Decreased coherence.
   C. Increase in beta activity.
   D. Increase in dominant alpha frequency.
   E. Change most frequently seen in the high-frequency band.

4.4   EEG findings in delirium would include

   A. Slowing.
   B. Quantitative EEG signal correlated with severity and duration of delirium.
   C. The finding that slowing cannot be meaningfully used in a patient with concomitant dementia.
   D. A and C.
   E. A and B.

4.5   Regarding seizures in the elderly, which of the following is true?

    A. Incidence is quite low.
    B. Approximately half are related to either strokes or tumors.
    C. Seizures rarely become recurrent.
    D. These patients would not be expected to demonstrate a normal EEG.
    E. Alzheimer's disease is rarely a risk factor.

4.6   The P3 evoked potential wave

    A. Is thought to reflect processes related to attention and immediate memory.
    B. Increases in latency with age in normal subjects.
    C. Increases in latency only in patients with dementia.
    D. Is distinguishable between subtypes of cortical dementias.
    E. A and B.

4.7   Within normal aging

    A. Approximately 30%–50% of elders show no evidence of cortical atrophy, cell loss, senile neuritic plaques, or neurofibrillary tangles.
    B. Neuritic plaques or neurofibrillary tangles are not observed.
    C. Distributional frequency of neuritic plaques consistently correlates with cognitive function.
    D. Neurofibrillary tangle frequency and distribution do not predict cognitive function.
    E. None of the above.

4.8   Alzheimer's disease is associated with which of the following?

    A. Hirano bodies.
    B. Granulovacuolar degeneration.
    C. Asymmetrical atrophy and brain weight loss.
    D. A and B.
    E. A and C.

4.9   Dementia with Lewy bodies includes all of the following neuropathological correlates *except*

    A. Neurofibrillary tangles.
    B. Neuritic plaques.
    C. More Lewy bodies in the substantia nigra than in idiopathic Parkinson's disease.
    D. Alpha-synuclein expressed in Lewy bodies.
    E. Weight of the brain typically less than the weight of the brain of the patient with Alzheimer's disease.

Chapter 5

Chemical Messengers

Select the single best response for each question.

5.1   Cholinergic neurons have been shown

   A. To be major targets of degeneration in Alzheimer's disease.
   B. To be innervated by hypertrophied galanin terminals in Alzheimer's disease.
   C. To have large increases in the activity and number of high-affinity choline uptake transporter sites in Alzheimer's disease.
   D. A, B, and C.
   E. A and C.

5.2   Changes of aging that occur in dopamine and dopamine receptors include

   A. Decreased numbers of D_2 receptors in the striatum with increasing age correlated with decreased cognitive function.
   B. Decreased dopamine transporter in caudate/putamen in oldest subjects.
   C. Correlation with decreased glucose metabolism of the frontal, temporal, and cingulate cortices.
   D. A, B, and C.
   E. None of the above.

5.3   Serotonergic neurons

   A. Do not show alterations of tryptophan hydroxylase with increasing age.
   B. Show a 10% increase per decade in binding of 5-HT_{1A}.
   C. Show a 17% increase per decade of 5-HT_{2A} receptors.
   D. Increase the serotonin transporter number in the striatum.
   E. None of the above.

5.4   Brain corticotropin-releasing factor (CRF) concentrations are noted to be

   A. Increased in frontal and temporal cortex of postmortem brains of patients with Alzheimer's disease compared to controls.
   B. Increased in nucleus basalis and hypothalamus in patients with Alzheimer's disease.
   C. Either unchanged, increased, or decreased in cerebrospinal fluid (CSF) from subjects with Alzheimer's disease, depending on the study cited.
   D. Poor diagnostic markers of dementia severity in Alzheimer's disease.
   E. None of the above.

5.5   Which of the following statements is true?

   A. Somatostatin and acetylcholine changes in Alzheimer's disease occur sometime after CRF loss.
   B. Nitric oxide has been hypothesized to contribute to oxidative damage at the cellular level in Alzheimer's disease.
   C. Somatostatin levels may increase with age.
   D. A and B.
   E. A, B, and C.

Chapter 6

Genetics

Select the single best response for each question.

6.1   The following are all examples of genes on which loci for Alzheimer's disease are found *except*

      A. Chromosome 1.
      B. Chromosome 14.
      C. Chromosome 19.
      D. Chromosome 21.
      E. Chromosome 24.

6.2   Which of the following statements is true of purported loci, genes, and mutations associated with Alzheimer's disease?

      A. The pathogenic mechanisms of *APP*, *PS1*, and *PS2* mutations are completely understood.
      B. Mutations appear to be associated with decreased production of the long form of beta-amyloid.
      C. Mutations appear to be associated with increased production of the short form of beta-amyloid.
      D. The short form of beta-amyloid is less pathogenic than the long form.
      E. The long form of beta-amyloid is less pathogenic than the short form.

6.3   Frontotemporal dementia (FTD) has been the focus of genetic investigations in recent years because approximately what percentage of those with FTD have a family history of the disorder?

      A. 20%.
      B. 30%.
      C. 40%.
      D. 50%.
      E. 70%.

6.4   In Parkinson's disease, genetics point to which of the following?

      A. Some evidence indicates that, parallel to Alzheimer's disease, age at onset is inherited.
      B. Replication studies have consistently confirmed candidate genes under study.
      C. Genes identified to date have dissimilar mechanisms of action.
      D. Ubiquitin proteasome pathway is not thought to be figurative in cell death.
      E. The mode of inheritance appears to be similar among the loci.

6.5 Genetics of depression in the elderly include all of the following *except*

A. More men of a depressed group with short alleles of the serotonin transporter–linked polymorphic region *(5HTTLPR)* as compared to controls.

B. Those elderly with short alleles showed a more rapid reduction in Hamilton Rating Scale for Depression when treated with paroxetine, as compared to those with long alleles.

C. Depressed elderly individuals carrying at least one *APOE* epsilon 4 had white matter intensities on MRI scans.

D. There is an association between subcortical gray matter hyperintensities and presence of at least one *APOE* epsilon 4 allele.

E. There has not been a consistent relation between *APOE* epsilon 4 allele and late-life depression.

Chapter 7

Psychological Aspects of Normal Aging

Select the single best response for each question.

7.1 Memory aging research has shown that

    A. Age-related declines tend to increase as the environmental support provided by the task decreases.

    B. Age-related declines are more evident in recall tasks than in recognition tasks.

    C. Significant age-related decline occurs in the capacity of primary memory.

    D. A and B.

    E. A, B, and C.

7.2 Communication abilities of older adults show all of the following changes *except*

    A. Substantial age-related deficits in discourse, text, or prose processing.

    B. Level of education and verbal intelligence could account for some portion of the observed age effect on text recall performance.

    C. Traditional laboratory-based problem-solving tasks do not seem to be predictive of everyday problem-solving performances for older adults.

    D. Older adults have been shown to have deficits in auditory processing in laboratory settings.

    E. Older adults do not seem to have disproportionate problems in processing everyday conversations or spoken input from television or radio.

7.3 Neuroimaging studies of normal older adults show

    A. Preferential deterioration of right-hemisphere structures.

    B. Generalized brain atrophy and decreases in resting cerebral blood flow with advanced age.

    C. Demyelination of subcortical, periventricular brain structures is rare in aging.

    D. No selective frontal lobe decline in the aging brain.

    E. Unchanged frontal lobe blood flow.

7.4 Research on intellectual functioning has shown which of the following?

    A. Fluid abilities tend to remain stable over the adult life span.

    B. Cognition and functional capacities are not closely related.

    C. Alzheimer's disease is projected to quadruple every 5 years after age 65.

    D. Studies from around the world have shown that about a quarter to a third of living centenarians may have dementia.

    E. Compared with other illnesses such as type II diabetes or diastolic hypertension, age itself is the strongest predictor of performing at or below the twenty-fifth percentile on a battery of neuropsychological tests.

7.5   Regarding the personality structure of the elderly,

   A. It has been shown to have remarkable stability over long periods of the life span.
   B. There are declines on dimensions of neuroticism.
   C. There are increases on dimensions of openness to experience.
   D. A and B.
   E. A and C.

7.6   Which of the following is *not* true of coping in later life?

   A. Older people have lower levels of internal control.
   B. Religious affiliation and strong spiritual beliefs serve to offset and buffer negative effects of some life experiences.
   C. Minority groups express greater satisfaction in using religion as a coping strategy.
   D. Religious beliefs and practices could be related to lower levels of depression.
   E. Older persons have less emotional reactivity when faced with stress than do younger adults.

7.7   Research on caregiving has shown that

   A. Depression and burden are higher among white caregivers than among African American caregivers.
   B. Depression and burden are higher among white caregivers than among Hispanic caregivers.
   C. Telephone interventions are not particularly effective for elderly persons.
   D. African American caregivers tend to use less positive appraisal than white caregivers.
   E. African American caregivers who appraised greater caregiving rewards were most likely to have higher levels of education.

Chapter 8

Social and Economic Factors Related to Psychiatric Disorders in Late Life

Select the single best response for each question.

8.1   Evidence concerning the relation between race and psychiatric morbidity of the elderly demonstrates that

  A. Race differences in depressive symptoms among the elderly are clear-cut.
  B. Older Hispanics appear to report higher levels of depressive symptoms than do whites or African Americans.
  C. There is a higher prevalence of alcohol and drug abuse among whites.
  D. There is a consistently higher level of depressive symptoms in African Americans than among whites.
  E. None of the above.

8.2   In general, all of the following are true *except*

  A. High levels of psychiatric symptoms are strongly related to low levels of education.
  B. Socioeconomic status and education in particular are weaker predictors of psychiatric symptoms in late life than at younger ages.
  C. Retirement increases the risk of psychiatric disorders.
  D. Women who have been widowed more than once are at greater risk for depression than those widowed only once.
  E. No evidence indicates that childbearing history is related to psychiatric status during later life.

8.3   Church attendance and participation in other religious activities are associated with a decreased risk of

  A. Alcohol abuse.
  B. Depression.
  C. Anxiety.
  D. A and B.
  E. A, B, and C.

8.4   Risk factors for psychiatric disorders in late life include all of the following *except*

  A. Chronic physical illnesses.
  B. Cognitive impairment.
  C. Perceived poor health.
  D. Disability as measured in terms of activities of daily living impairment.
  E. Lack of substantial social network size.

8.5   Recovery from depression is

A. Affected by the presence of a confidant.
B. Affected by social network size.
C. Affected by perception of high-quality support.
D. Unrelated to religious participation.
E. More strongly predicted by the clinical features of the index episode than by social factors.

8.6   Among older alcoholics, more favorable outcomes were associated with

A. Female gender.
B. Higher socioeconomic status.
C. White race.
D. Being married, especially among men.
E. All of the above.

8.7   Mental health service use by the elderly has shown all of the following *except*

A. Women are more likely to seek care for psychiatric problems.
B. Gender is related to volume of care received.
C. Older patients, ages 65 and older, are less likely to seek mental health treatment than those ages 25–64.
D. Only age is a significant predictor of both receipt and volume of care.
E. Need factors are not significant predictors of volume of care received.

8.8   Which of the following statements about older adults seeking outpatient care for mental health problems is true?

A. Most receive diagnoses and treatment in the general medical sector.
B. Older adults are far less likely than the middle aged to receive mental health treatment from psychiatrists.
C. Eighty percent of all older adults with primary or secondary psychiatric diagnoses receive treatment by primary care physicians.
D. A and B.
E. A, B, and C.

Chapter 9

The Psychiatric Interview of Older Adults

Select the single best response for each question.

9.1　The psychiatric interview of older adults can be complicated by

　　A.　Their not equating present distress with past episodes that are symptomatically similar.
　　B.　Their becoming angry or irritated when a clinician continues to probe previous periods of overt disability in usual activities.
　　C.　Their having experienced a major illness or trauma in childhood but viewing this information as being of no relevance to the present episode.
　　D.　A histrionic personality style.
　　E.　All of the above.

9.2　Medication history of the older adult

　　A.　Should involve having the older person bring in all pill bottles.
　　B.　Should involve a double check between the written schedule and pill containers.
　　C.　Should assess alcohol intake.
　　D.　Should assess substance abuse.
　　E.　All of the above.

9.3　Evaluation of the family of the psychiatrically ill older adult would include all of the following parameters of support *except*

　　A.　Availability of the family member.
　　B.　Tangible services provided by the family.
　　C.　Patient's perception of family support.
　　D.　Tolerance by the family of specific behaviors derived from the psychiatric disorder.
　　E.　Consideration of only those individuals genetically related to the patient.

9.4　Examples of depressive delusions would be least likely to involve which of the following statements?

　　A.　"I've lost my mind."
　　B.　"My body is disintegrating."
　　C.　"I ought to be executed."
　　D.　"I have an incurable illness."
　　E.　"I have caused some great harm."

9.5 Barriers to effective communication between the older patient and clinician can include

A. Physician perceiving the older adult patient incorrectly because of personal fears of aging and death.
B. The patient's perceptual problems.
C. Patient taking longer to respond to inquiries, resisting the physician who attempts to hurry through the interview.
D. Patient perceiving the physician unrealistically.
E. All of the above.

Chapter 10

Use of the Laboratory in the Diagnostic Workup of Older Adults

Select the single best response for each question.

10.1 Serum vitamin B_{12} and folate levels

    A. Are rarely important in the evaluation of the elderly patient.

    B. May point to etiologies of a range of neuropsychiatric disturbances.

    C. Would not be thought etiologic if recorded as normal.

    D. Are not related to hyperhomocysteinemia.

    E. Are not related to one-carbon metabolism in brain tissue.

10.2 Approximately what percentage of persons admitted from the community to a geropsychiatry unit may have a urinary tract infection that may result in a delirium?

    A. 10%.

    B. 20%.

    C. 35%.

    D. 45%.

    E. 55%.

10.3 Lithium is most likely to demonstrate which of the following ECG changes?

    A. AV block.

    B. Prolonged PR interval.

    C. Sick sinus syndrome.

    D. Bradycardia.

    E. QTc prolongation.

10.4 *APOE* testing has shown that

    A. A homozygous epsilon 4/epsilon 4 genotype is diagnostic for Alzheimer's disease.

    B. It is valuable in modifying the disease course and influencing current supportive treatments for Alzheimer's disease.

    C. It predicts response to cholinesterase inhibitors.

    D. It lacks hierarchy of the alleles for prediction or risk for development of Alzheimer's disease.

    E. None of the above.

10.5 Which of the following statements about genetic testing is *not* true? Genetic testing

    A. Results in transient heightened anxiety and depression.
    B. Can possibly result in hopelessness.
    C. Results in job loss or lack of insurability.
    D. Proves to be a valuable tool with untapped potential.
    E. Is recommended to predict dementia risk in asymptomatic individuals.

10.6 Differences between AIDS-related and Alzheimer's dementia include all of the following *except*

    A. Mild protein elevation of CSF in Alzheimer's disease.
    B. Mononuclear CSF pleocytosis in AIDS-related dementia.
    C. Neuropathies in AIDS-related dementia.
    D. Aphasia and other cortical deficits uncommon in AIDS-related dementia.
    E. Cortical dementia in Alzheimer's disease.

Chapter 11

Neuropsychological Assessment of Dementia

Select the single best response for each question.

11.1   The most common cause for cognitive change after age 50 is

    A. Alzheimer's disease.
    B. Frontotemporal dementia.
    C. Normal aging of the nervous system.
    D. Vascular dementia.
    E. None of the above.

11.2   The differences underlying memory loss of normal aging and that of Alzheimer's disease include

    A. Consolidation or storage of new information in long-term memory stores.
    B. Efficient accessing of recently stored information.
    C. Difficulty with visuospatial tasks.
    D. A and B.
    E. A, B, and C.

11.3   The leading cause of dementia in elderly persons is

    A. Vascular disease.
    B. Alzheimer's disease.
    C. Lewy body disease.
    D. Frontotemporal disease.
    E. Corticobasal degeneration.

11.4   The earliest manifestation of Alzheimer's disease is

    A. Rapid forgetting of new information after very brief delays.
    B. Expressive language difficulty.
    C. Visuospatial difficulty.
    D. Apraxia.
    E. Circumlocution.

11.5   Patients with vascular dementia could be expected to show all of the following *except*

   A. Memory deficits often patchy in nature.
   B. Impaired recollection of some recent event but surprisingly good memory of some other event occurring during the same time frame.
   C. Flattened learning curve over repeated trials.
   D. Low recall performance as well as rapid forgetting.
   E. Recognition improving dramatically with a recognition format.

11.6   The frontal variant of frontotemporal dementia would be expected to manifest

   A. Mutism.
   B. Preservation of insight.
   C. Recent memory impairment.
   D. Changes in social behavior and personality.
   E. Complaint of word loss and restriction in expressive vocabulary.

11.7   What percentage of patients with Parkinson's disease are reported to have dementia?

   A. 5%–10%.
   B. 10%–20%.
   C. 20%–40%.
   D. 50%–60%.
   E. 70%–80%.

11.8   Geriatric depression shows all of the following deficits *except*

   A. Impairments on tests sensitive to frontal lobe function.
   B. Difficulties on sustained and selective attention.
   C. Set shifting.
   D. Perseverative errors and intrusional tendencies.
   E. All cognitive impairments remitting with treatment.

Chapter 12

Cognitive Disorders

Select the single best response for each question.

12.1   Computed tomography (CT) and magnetic resonance imaging (MRI) can detect which of the following as potentially treatable causes of dementia?

    A. Tumors.
    B. Subdural hematomas.
    C. Periventricular hyperintensities on T2-weighted images.
    D. A and B.
    E. A, B, and C.

12.2   Cognitive deficits of Alzheimer's disease correlate

    A. With density of neurofibrillary tangles.
    B. With hyperphosphorylated tau.
    C. With density of neuritic plaques.
    D. A and B.
    E. A and C.

12.3   Serotonin abnormalities of Alzheimer's disease include

    A. Loss of serotonergic neurons in brain stem raphe nuclei.
    B. Decreased concentration of serotonin in brain tissue.
    C. Decreased concentration of serotonin in CSF.
    D. Decreased serotonin receptor concentrations.
    E. All of the above.

12.4   Brain presynaptic cholinergic deficit has *not* been demonstrated in which of the following?

    A. Alzheimer's disease.
    B. Frontotemporal dementia.
    C. Vascular dementia.
    D. Lewy body dementia.
    E. C and D.

12.5   Cholinesterase inhibitors are best conceptualized as drugs

    A. That stabilize cognition, activities of daily living, and behavioral function.
    B. That improve cognitive function greatly.
    C. Only indicated for mild to moderate stages of Alzheimer's disease.
    D. Contraindicated in the treatment of Lewy body dementia.
    E. Predominately associated with the side effect of sedation.

12.6 Vitamin E and selegiline have *not* been shown to

   A. Have beneficial effects on cognitive function per se.
   B. Delay nursing home placement.
   C. Delay progression to severe dementia.
   D. Be more effective in combination than either agent alone.
   E. Delay loss of basic activities of daily living.

12.7 Dementia with a cerebrovascular contribution

   A. Is as common as Alzheimer's disease.
   B. Is most frequently seen as pure vascular dementia.
   C. Lowers the threshold for and increases the magnitude of dementia caused by Alzheimer's disease.
   D. Is associated with an especially high prevalence and severity of dementia with infarcts in the basal ganglia, thalamus, or deep white matter.
   E. C and D.

12.8 Most forms of frontotemporal dementia involve

   A. Neuronal cell loss.
   B. Gliosis.
   C. Pick bodies.
   D. Abnormal function of tau protein.
   E. Amyloidopathy.

12.9 Hypothyroidism

   A. Can produce a dementia accompanied by irritability, paranoid ideation, and depression.
   B. Can produce a dementia for which aggressive thyroid replacement results in the patient's return to previous level of functioning.
   C. Is similar to vitamin B_{12} deficiency dementia in that B_{12} replacement leads to remission of dementia.
   D. A and B.
   E. A, B, and C.

12.10 Delirium in the elderly

   A. Usually persists for months in those hospitalized for medical or surgical reasons.
   B. Rarely results in full resolution of symptoms in a short time.
   C. Is often the initial presentation of an underlying dementia.
   D. Could have an insidious onset.
   E. All of the above.

Chapter 13

Movement Disorders

Select the single best response for each question.

13.1   All of the following are features of Parkinson's disease *except*

   A. Postural instability.
   B. Prevalence increasing with age.
   C. Lewy bodies in the cytoplasm of degenerating neurons.
   D. Resting tremor attenuating at least transiently during voluntary movement, much like that of essential tremor.
   E. Presentation with an akinetic form in which resting tremor is minimal.

13.2   Synkinetic movement refers to

   A. Resting tremor.
   B. Cogwheel rigidity.
   C. Involuntary resistance to passive movement of the extremities.
   D. Voluntary movement of contralateral extremity bringing out rigidity in ipsilateral limb.
   E. None of the above.

13.3   Side effects of dopamine agonists include which of the following?

   A. Hallucinations.
   B. Dyskinesias.
   C. Dystonia.
   D. A and B.
   E. A, B, and C.

13.4   All of the following are features of progressive supranuclear palsy (PSP) *except*

   A. Vertical gaze palsy.
   B. Early postural instability.
   C. Axial rigidity greater than appendicular rigidity.
   D. Good response to levodopa.
   E. Sloppy eating.

13.5   Which of the following is *not* true of essential tremor?

   A. It is the most prevalent movement disorder among the elderly.
   B. Prevalence increases with age.
   C. Frequency may decrease with age.
   D. Early on, tremor is absent at rest.
   E. Usually it is not associated with a family history of tremor.

13.6 Which of the following attenuates essential tremor?

    A. Propranolol.
    B. Primidone.
    C. Alcohol.
    D. Deep brain stimulation of the ventral intermediate nucleus of the contralateral thalamus.
    E. All of the above.

C h a p t e r   1 4

Mood Disorders

Select the single best response for each question.

14.1   In contrast to low rates of major depression among older adults in the community, it has been estimated that up to what percentage of hospitalized elders fulfill criteria for a major depressive episode?

    A. 6%.
    B. 11%.
    C. 16%.
    D. 21%.
    E. 31%.

14.2   Mortality among elderly patients is

    A. Increased in older men with physical health problems and depression.
    B. Increased among nursing home patients with depression.
    C. Increased in previously hospitalized depressed women.
    D. A and B.
    E. A, B, and C.

14.3   Studies of prognosis of late-life depression show all of the following *except*

    A. Older adults differ from their middle-age counterparts in terms of recovery and remission.
    B. Elders who have recovered appear to experience residual depressive symptoms.
    C. Seventy percent of elderly patients with major depression treated with adequate antidepressant regimens recover from the index episode.
    D. Older patients who have experienced one or more moderate to severe episodes of major depression may need to continue antidepressant therapy permanently to minimize relapse.
    E. Physical illness and cognitive impairment are associated with a worse outcome.

14.4   Bipolar disorder in the elderly may have all of the following characteristics *except*

    A. Tendency toward more rapid recurrences late in the illness.
    B. Stressful events more likely to precede early-onset mania than late-onset mania.
    C. Increased cerebral vulnerability playing a stronger role than life events in precipitating late-onset mania.
    D. Association with low rates of familial affective disorder.
    E. Genetic factors weighing heavily in the etiology.

14.5   Late-onset psychotic depression is characterized by which of the following?

A. Individuals with delusional depression tend to be older and respond to ECT.
B. Delusions of guilt are more common than delusions of persecution or of having an incurable illness.
C. It is not associated with poor social support.
D. Focus on the abdomen is uncommon.
E. None of the above.

14.6   Uncomplicated bereavement is usually considered to include virtually all symptoms of depression, with the exception of _____, and to last up to _____ months.

A. Extreme feelings of worthlessness, 2 months.
B. Extreme feelings of worthlessness, 6 months.
C. Irritability and hostility, 2 months.
D. Irritability and hostility, 6 months.
E. Sensations of somatic distress, 6 months.

14.7   Reversible dementia due to depression

A. Predicts poor response to treatment of the depression.
B. Is associated with patients attempting to conceal disabilities rather than highlighting them on formal mental status exam.
C. Cannot be differentiated from that of bona fide dementia by way of REM sleep measures.
D. Often indicates the presence of an early dementing illness.
E. Should not be treated with a potent anticholinergic antidepressant such as imipramine.

14.8   According to a recent study, what percentage of elders fulfill criteria for definite or questionable alcohol abuse?

A. Between 2% and 4%.
B. Between 3% and 6%.
C. Between 10% and 15%.
D. Between 20% and 30%.
E. Between 30% and 40%.

14.9   ECT

A. Is less effective in older adults than in younger ones.
B. Is no more effective than and has more side effects than antidepressants when used in the old-old populace.
C. Has a relapse rate that may exceed 50% in the year after a course of ECT, without prophylaxis.
D. Leads to a significant worsening of cognition in the majority of elderly depressed patients with dementia.
E. Should be avoided in patients with cardiovascular, neurological, endocrine, or metabolic conditions.

Chapter 15

Schizophrenia and Paranoid Disorders

Select the single best response for each question.

15.1 Factors distinguishing patients with very late onset schizophrenia from "true" schizophrenia of younger patients include all of the following *except*

A. Lower genetic load.
B. Less evidence of early childhood maladjustment.
C. Relative lack of formal thought disorder and negative symptoms.
D. Lesser risk of tardive dyskinesia.
E. Evidence of a neurodegenerative rather than a neurodevelopmental process.

15.2 What approximate percentage of Alzheimer's disease patients manifest psychotic symptoms, typically in the middle stages of the disease?

A. 10%–20%.
B. 15%–25%.
C. 25%–30%.
D. 35%–50%.
E. 55%–65%.

15.3 Alzheimer's disease patients with and without psychosis differ in all of the following *except*

A. Alzheimer's disease patients with psychosis show greater impairment in executive functioning.
B. Alzheimer's disease patients with psychosis have a greater prevalence of extrapyramidal signs.
C. Alzheimer's disease patients with psychosis have shown increased norepinephrine levels and reduced serotonin levels in subcortical regions.
D. Alzheimer's disease patients with psychosis typically warrant very long term maintenance therapy with antipsychotics.
E. Alzheimer's disease patients with psychosis have more prevalent behavioral disturbances such as agitation than hallucinations and paranoid delusions.

15.4 Patients with dementia with Lewy bodies could be safely treated with all of the following *except*

A. Donepezil.
B. Quetiapine.
C. Rivastigmine.
D. Olanzapine.
E. Clozapine.

15.5 The most important risk factor for tardive dyskinesia is

    A. Alcohol abuse.
    B. Early extrapyramidal symptoms.
    C. Certain ethnicities.
    D. Aging.
    E. None of the above.

Chapter 16

Anxiety and Panic Disorders

Select the single best response for each question.

16.1 According to the Epidemiologic Catchment Area (ECA) study of the 1980s, the combined prevalence of phobia, panic disorder, and obsessive-compulsive disorder in people over age 65 is approximately what percentage?

A. 2.5%.
B. 3.5%.
C. 5.5%.
D. 6.5%.
E. 7%.

16.2 Panic disorder in those older than 65

A. Has a point prevalence of 0.4%.
B. Is not uncommonly ascribed to other causes by the elderly.
C. May present with fewer symptoms.
D. Is a relatively uncommon development in late life.
E. All of the above.

16.3 In at least one study, what percentage of elderly Holocaust survivors met criteria for posttraumatic stress disorder more than 40 years after the war?

A. 10%.
B. 20%.
C. 30%.
D. 40%.
E. 50%.

16.4 The most common anxiety disorder of the elderly population is

A. Generalized anxiety disorder.
B. Posttraumatic stress disorder.
C. Social phobia.
D. Specific phobia.
E. Obsessive-compulsive disorder.

16.5 Which of the following factors could pertain to medical illnesses and anxiety among the elderly?

A. The older adult may worry about the effect and meaning of physical illness.
B. Anxiety may contribute to medical problems and complications.
C. Many anxiety symptoms may masquerade as medical illness.
D. Anxiety symptoms may be caused by medications given to elderly persons.
E. All of the above.

16.6 Which of the following pharmacological agents has become the mainstay treatment of anxiety disorder in the elderly?

    A. Tricyclic antidepressants (TCAs).
    B. Monoamine oxidase inhibitors (MAOIs).
    C. Selective serotonin reuptake inhibitors (SSRIs).
    D. Benzodiazepines.
    E. Buspirone.

Chapter 17

Somatoform Disorders

Select the single best response for each question.

17.1 Somatization disorder is a psychiatric illness characterized by numerous physical complaints that are in excess of examination findings. This may be an especially challenging problem in the older patient with other chronic medical conditions. Which of the following is also true regarding somatization disorder?

A. Paralleling the relative risk for depressive disorders, the risk for somatization disorder in women is twice that in men.

B. Somatization disorder is common in patients with irritable bowel disease.

C. As somatization disorder patients age, their reported symptoms tend to change and symptoms are reported in a less consistent pattern.

D. Prominent pain symptoms are the typical "pseudoneurological" presentation.

E. Another term for somatization disorder is Munchausen syndrome.

17.2 Undifferentiated somatoform disorder and hypochondriasis may present in the geriatric psychiatric patient. Distinguishing between these two conditions may be difficult in the clinical setting. Which of the following statements is true?

A. Undifferentiated somatoform disorder requires the presence of persistent physical complaints for at least 12 months.

B. Patients with chronic pain rarely also qualify for a diagnosis of undifferentiated somatoform disorder.

C. The psychological preoccupation in hypochondriasis relates to the symptoms experienced, rather than the possible disease "represented" by the symptoms.

D. It has been clearly established that high educational level and high socioeconomic status lead to a predisposition to hypochondriasis, because individuals with these factors may be more aware of medical conditions and have greater access to information.

E. Comorbid depressive and anxiety disorders are common in hypochondriasis.

17.3 Conversion disorder is characterized by motor and/or sensory deficits that suggest neurological illness(es) but that cannot be elucidated by the appropriate neurological and neuroimaging evaluations. Which of the following is true regarding this syndrome?

A. Conversion disorder is more common in elderly than in young patients.

B. Conversion disorder is seen almost exclusively in women.

C. Comorbidity in conversion disorder includes substance abuse and head injury.

D. Although nonepileptic seizures (often referred to as pseudoseizures) are a subtype of conversion disorder, they are rarely seen in patients with a bona fide seizure disorder.

E. As with younger patients, elderly patients with conversion disorder infrequently have an "actual" comorbid neurological disorder.

17.4 Pain is a common complaint in geriatric medicine; therefore, appreciation of the psychiatric aspects of pain disorders is important for the physician treating these patients. Which of the following is true of pain disorders?

A. Alzheimer's disease may lower the pain threshold, thus altering the pain perception in these patients.

B. In patients with chronic low back pain, psychiatric comorbidity typically follows the onset of the chronic pain syndrome.

C. Specific descriptions of pain due solely to psychological factors can be readily distinguished from pain states where there is an "obvious" general medical condition.

D. In the Okasha et al. (1999) study on headache, somatoform pain disorder was twice as common in the nonorganic-etiology group as in the organic-etiology group.

E. In the Aigner and Bach (1999) study on chronic pain, hypochondriasis was the most common comorbid somatoform disorder.

17.5 The etiology of somatoform disorders has been subject to much theoretical speculation. Which of the following is true?

A. The prevalence of all definitively diagnosed somatoform disorders increases with age.

B. When somatoform disorders present in the older patient, comorbid neurological illness may be associated with them, but neuropsychological (cognitive) impairment is not.

C. Somatoform disorders are associated with a history of serious illness of a parent, but not in the patient, early in life.

D. Comorbid panic disorder is common in somatoform disorders, but other anxiety disorders are not.

E. The personality trait of neuroticism, wherein the subject experiences more negative emotions, is associated with the development of somatoform disorders.

17.6 Treatment of somatoform disorders calls for an integrative biopsychosocial approach by the physician. Which of the following approaches is recommended?

A. The physician should arrange appointments on an as-needed basis.

B. A focus on obtaining insight into the psychological context of somatoform symptoms should be the first priority for intervention.

C. The physician should not offer to review all prior medical records, as this merely reinforces maladaptive somatization behavior.

D. Hypochondriasis has been shown to respond to antidepressants and anxiolytics.

E. Hypnosis should be avoided in conversion disorder as these patients are rarely subject to induction of hypnosis.

Chapter 18

Sexual Disorders

Select the single best response for each question.

18.1 Sexual function in older patients may be an important area of quality of life and needs thoughtful and sensitive clinical assessment. Which of the following statements is true regarding the Jacoby (1999) study of late-life sexuality?

  A. The study involved face-to-face interviews.
  B. Subjects ranged in age from 55 to 80.
  C. Among respondents over age 75, men were three times as likely as women to have a steady sexual partner.
  D. The majority of subjects of both sexes stated that sexual activity was important to their quality of life.
  E. About 50% of respondents remained sexually active.

18.2 Masters and Johnson's groundbreaking research (1966) described the human sexual response in a four-stage model, each stage corresponding with specific psychological and/or physiological events. Which of the following stages is not included in Masters and Johnson's model?

  A. Desire.
  B. Excitement or arousal.
  C. Plateau.
  D. Orgasm.
  E. Resolution.

18.3 Sexual function is affected by aging and is thus an issue of great interest to the geropsychiatrist. Which of the following statements is true regarding sexual function and age?

  A. In men, testosterone levels decrease notably beginning at age 50.
  B. Erectile dysfunction affects more than 50% of men ages 40 to 70.
  C. Erectile dysfunction affects more than 95% of men over age 70.
  D. Among older women, dyspareunia is common, but hypoactive sexual desire disorder is infrequent.
  E. Impaired arousal due to diabetic vascular disease is an example of a secondary effect on sexual function.

18.4 Medications are a common cause of sexual dysfunction in older patients. Which of the following is *not* true regarding various compensatory strategies physicians can consider to address this problem?

  A. Continue medication while tolerance to the medication develops, after which sexual function may spontaneously improve.
  B. Reduce dose to a level without sexual side effects.
  C. Try a drug holiday for a medication with a long half-life.
  D. Simplify a complex regimen of medications.
  E. Switch to an alternative medication with less risk of sexual side effects.

18.5 Unfortunately, antidepressant medications (particularly selective serotonin reuptake inhibitors [SSRIs]) have been associated with sexual dysfunction as a medication-induced side effect. There are several antidotes that the psychiatrist can use to address this problem. However, the subsequent loss of primary antidepressant effect is a concerning possibility. Which of the following antidotes can reverse the antidepressant effect of SSRIs?

A. Yohimbine.
B. Amantadine.
C. Cyproheptadine.
D. Bethanecol.
E. Methylphenidate.

18.6 Erectile dysfunction (ED) is the most common sexual dysfunction in male patients, and its risk increases with age. Which of the following is true regarding the genesis and management of ED?

A. Erectile physiology is implicated in less than 50% of cases of ED.
B. Hypogonadism with resultant testosterone deficiency should be treated with exogenous testosterone, even in cases of prostate cancer.
C. Sildenafil (Viagra) is effective only in men with ED due to "organic" causes.
D. Spontaneous erections (without physical stimulation) often follow dosing of sildenafil.
E. Side effects of sildenafil include headache, flushing, gastrointestinal discomfort, and blurred vision.

18.7 Inappropriate sexual behavior in dementia may cause great disruption to caregivers and institutions managing care for these patients and thus requires effective intervention. Which of the following is *not* true regarding problematic sexual behavior in dementia?

A. Inappropriate sexual behavior in dementia is seen in 25% of cases, whether patients are in the community or institutionalized.
B. Caregivers and staff should set verbal limits and redirect sexually inappropriate behaviors of patients with dementia.
C. Restrictive clothing may be used to minimize incidents of genital display and self-stimulation.
D. Excess libidinal urges in dementia can be treated by SSRI or beta-blocker.
E. Estrogen can be used to decrease sexual aggression in male patients with dementia.

Chapter 19

Bereavement and Adjustment Disorders

Select the single best response for each question.

19.1 Bereavement is a common focus of clinical inquiry in geropsychiatry. The epidemiology of partner loss as a locus for bereavement has led to some conclusions that are of interest to the practicing clinician. Which of the following is true regarding widowhood and widowerhood in the United States?

    A. The mean age of spousal loss is 3 years older for women than for men.

    B. The mean duration of widowhood for women is twice that of widowerhood for men.

    C. The rates of widowhood among persons older than 65 are much higher for Hispanic and Asian Americans than for Caucasians.

    D. Among those older than 65, women are twice as likely as men (30% vs. 15%) to have lost a spouse.

    E. Following the loss of a spouse, women are at a higher risk for mortality than are men.

19.2 Numerous theories of attachment have been posited and applied to the clinical problem of bereavement. Which of the following is true?

    A. Bowlby's attachment theory holds that separation anxiety and pining serve to facilitate emotional withdrawal from the lost object.

    B. In accordance with theories of adaptation, grief symptoms typically abate in elderly widows and widowers.

    C. Bowlby (1980) found that preoccupation with the lost spouse 12 months after his or her death occurred only in a small minority of subjects.

    D. The survivor who maintains abstract rather then concrete ties with the lost partner is more likely to manifest healthy adaptation to loss.

    E. Survivors who maintain contact with the lost partner through special possessions of the deceased experience less psychological distress and grief-specific symptoms.

19.3 Stroebe and Schut are notable for their recent work on a dual-process model of bereavement. According to this model, which of the following is considered to be a restoration-oriented rather than a loss-oriented stressor?

    A. Emotional symptoms.

    B. Behavioral symptoms.

    C. New identity development.

    D. Physiological symptoms.

    E. Cognitive symptoms.

19.4 An application of the dual-process model of grief is to focus on specific tasks required of the survivor. These are grouped into two categories: grief tasks and restoration tasks. All of the following challenges are considered to be grief tasks *except*

A. Acceptance of the changed world.
B. Confrontation of the loss.
C. Restructuring thoughts.
D. Restructuring memories.
E. Emotional withdrawal from the deceased without forgetting him or her.

19.5 Studies of ethnic and cultural differences in end-of-life and bereavement issues have revealed distinctions of clinical importance. Regarding Block's 1998 study of Latinos, particularly first- and second-generation, which of the following is *not* true?

A. Patients valued family input into treatment decisions.
B. Patients had extensive social networks.
C. Patients placed family interests above those of the self.
D. Patients resisted accepting death as unavoidable.
E. Patients preferred a caring rather than a scientific approach by the physician.

19.6 In clinical classification of cases that present with depressive symptoms in the context of interpersonal loss or grief, the physician often faces the task of deciding when symptoms cross the threshold of becoming complicated bereavement. This distinction is not always simple. To address this, DSM-IV-TR includes several specific symptoms that are not considered to be characteristic of a "normal" grief reaction. Which of the following symptoms would *not* be considered evidence of complicated bereavement?

A. Guilt about actions not taken at the time of death.
B. Preoccupation with personal worthlessness.
C. Marked psychomotor retardation.
D. Prolonged and marked functional impairment.
E. Hallucinations not containing imagery of the dead person.

19.7 Several longitudinal studies of late-life bereavement have revealed some specific findings. Which of the following is true?

A. Symptoms of anxiety and depression among bereaved subjects differ from controls only in the first 2 months following the loss.
B. All studies have shown a higher psychological symptom burden among bereaved men than among bereaved women.
C. When separated operationally from other symptoms such as anxiety and depression, grief has been found to remain for longer time periods.
D. Women have been found to have higher rates of persistent grief than men.
E. Older women who have lost their spouses have a higher risk of death than older bereaved men.

19.8   Which of the following is true regarding clinical interventions for complicated bereavement in older patients?

A. If depression is present, it should not be treated (specifically with medications) until the grieving process is addressed.

B. Even if major depression is present, it should not be treated for at least 4 months.

C. Since most deaths of elderly patients are due to chronic illness, posttraumatic stress disorder in survivors is rare.

D. Combined pharmacological and psychotherapeutic treatment has been shown to be more effective than either intervention alone.

E. The late-life depression research group in Pittsburgh (M.D. Miller et al. 1997; Reynolds et al. 1999), used fluoxetine as its antidepressant in research studies.

Chapter 20

Sleep and Circadian Rhythm Disorders

Select the single best response for each question.

20.1 Sleep disorders are an important and often obscure cause of clinical distress in elderly patients. As such, their full evaluation and thoughtful management may enhance patients' quality of life substantially. Which of the following is true?

    A. One-quarter of noninstitutionalized persons older than 65 report chronic sleep problems.

    B. Despite clinical distress due to sleep disorders, they are an infrequent reason for long-term care placement.

    C. Most age-related sleep disturbances are caused by primary, as opposed to secondary, sleep-related symptoms.

    D. Sleep and circadian rhythm changes in elderly patients are absent unless there is a sleep disorder.

    E. With increasing age, an increased number of arousals is causative in the increased amount of nocturnal wake time.

20.2 Sleep apnea (SA), periodic limb movement disorder (PLMD), and restless legs syndrome (RLS) are relatively commonly encountered in older patients. Which of the following is true?

    A. The more common form of SA in elderly patients is central rather than obstructive.

    B. SA, even in mild cases, is not associated with insomnia.

    C. The primary treatment of obstructive SA is surgical.

    D. Clinically significant PLMD is five to six times more common in elderly patients, when compared to younger adults.

    E. Polysomnography is required for the diagnosis of both PLMD and RLS.

20.3 Alzheimer's disease and Parkinson's disease are associated with many neuropsychiatric complications. Among these is disturbed sleep; when sleep disturbance is associated with behavioral agitation, the term "sundowning" is used. Which of the following is true regarding sleep disorders and their management in these neurodegenerative conditions?

    A. Alzheimer's disease patients have increased arousals and awakenings, and increased amounts of REM and slow-wave sleep.

    B. Benzodiazepines are the treatment of choice for the sundowning in Alzheimer's disease.

    C. Antipsychotics may be helpful for the treatment of Alzheimer's disease patients with sundowning, and the atypical agents are generally well tolerated.

    D. Sleep complaints are notable in less than one-half of Parkinson's disease patients.

    E. Although carbidopa/levodopa combinations may cause initial insomnia, they do not increase risk of nightmares.

20.4   Comorbid medical conditions are common in older patients with sleep complaints, and the management of the chronic illness may be of great utility in assisting these patients. Which of the following is true for those patients with chronic obstructive pulmonary disease (COPD)?

A. In COPD, the degree of sleep disruption is correlated with the degree of hypoxemia.
B. Daytime sleepiness is typical in COPD.
C. Polysomnography is routinely necessary to evaluate sleep complaints in COPD because sleep apnea is much more common in these patients.
D. Oral theophyllines are adenosine receptor antagonists and may themselves disrupt sleep in COPD.
E. Benzodiazepines are the treatment of choice for COPD patients with sleep complaints.

20.5   There are various methods by which to evaluate and classify sleep disorders. The patient who is suspected of having narcolepsy requires which of the following?

A. Polysomnography and multiple sleep latency test (MSLT).
B. Polysomnography and sleep log.
C. Actigraphy and sleep log.
D. Sleep log and MSLT.
E. Polysomnography and actigraphy.

20.6   Which of the following is true regarding treatment of sleep disorders?

A. The majority of sleep complaints are due to a primary sleep disorder, not an associated medical condition.
B. In patients with primary insomnia, medications are the first treatment option.
C. The most commonly prescribed hypnotic agents are atypical benzodiazepines.
D. Trazodone is FDA-approved for the short-term treatment of insomnia.
E. Zolpidem has the shortest half-life of the atypical benzodiazepines.

Chapter 21

Alcohol and Drug Problems

Select the single best response for each question.

21.1 Substance abuse and dependence problems may cause significant distress for the older patient and need to be evaluated fully by the geropsychiatrist. Which of the following is true regarding substance use disorders in this population?

A. The prevalence of substance use disorders in patients over 65 is roughly twice as high for men as for women.

B. Risk factors for elder substance abuse are similar to those for younger adults (e.g., male gender, lower educational attainment, and comorbid mood disorder).

C. Because alcohol is distributed to fatty tissues, older patients' higher body fat levels cause higher blood alcohol levels.

D. A major cause of greater psychoactive effects of alcohol on older patients is the age-related steady decrease in activity of alcohol dehydrogenase.

E. Alcohol leads to decreased sexual drive and impotence in male patients by an antiandrogen effect.

21.2 The physician may be consulted to manage some of the chronic effects of alcohol on neurophysiology and cognitive function in the elderly patient. Which of the following is true regarding alcohol's chronic effects?

A. Peripheral neuropathy in alcoholics, which often follows deficiency states of thiamine and other B-complex vitamins, is seen in 25% of chronic alcoholics.

B. The cognitive effects of alcohol typically result in a decreased overall level of intelligence as reflected in the IQ on formal testing.

C. Focal cognitive deficits with chronic alcoholism include deficits in visuospatial analysis and nonverbal abstraction.

D. End-stage alcoholic dementia features anterograde, but not retrograde, amnesia.

E. Alcoholic dementia deficits are permanent; abstinence does not reverse deficits in short-term memory.

21.3 Regarding the use of adjunctive medications to encourage abstinence and to facilitate recovery from alcohol dependence in elderly patents, which of the following is *not* true?

A. Disulfiram may be used, with due caution, in elderly patients.

B. Naltrexone is generally well tolerated in older patients.

C. The patient should be empowered to self-administer adjunctive medication.

D. Family members should be taught to lower their threshold for concern over even nondisruptive drinking by the patient.

E. Patients have been shown to increase compliance with treatment if family members are actively involved in treatment.

21.4   Abuse of or dependence on prescription medications is another common clinical problem in geriatric medicine. Which of the following is true?

A. Benzodiazepines represent approximately 20% of all medications prescribed for patients over 65.
B. Older women are twice as likely as older men to regularly use psychoactive drugs.
C. Older adults rarely share or swap prescribed medications with each other without telling their physicians.
D. Over-the-counter remedies are used nearly as frequently as prescribed medications by older patients.
E. In elderly patients, signs of lithium carbonate toxicity are unlikely if the serum level is below 1.0 mEq/L.

21.5   Which of the following is *not* true regarding alcohol use and older patients?

A. Alcohol use leads to increased mortality in midlife.
B. Among those who survive into old age, alcohol use continues to be associated with greater mortality.
C. Part of the reason for increased mortality in alcohol users is due to an increased risk of suicide.
D. The sleep in alcohol-dependent patients who are withdrawn from alcohol includes decreased REM sleep and increased slow-wave sleep.
E. When alcohol is used as a hypnotic, there is often a rebound awakening 4 hours into the sleep period.

21.6   The useful mnemonic **FRAMES** (Miller and Sanchez) can be used to organize clinical interventions for substance abuse in the elderly patient. Which of the following statements is *not* part of the **FRAMES** schema?

A. **F**eedback about substance use.
B. **R**esponsibility to address the problem of substance use.
C. **A**bstinence as an early requirement.
D. **M**enu of patient options.
E. **E**mpathy for the patient's ambivalence and challenge.

C h a p t e r 2 2

Personality Disorders

Select the single best response for each question.

22.1   Which of the following is true regarding personality disorders in older patients?

A. As research into personality disorders has increased, the phenomenon of personality disorders in the elderly has been thoroughly examined.

B. Unlike in younger patients, comorbid personality disorders in elderly patients do not appear to affect outcomes of mood disorders.

C. When an older patient's personality changes significantly due to dementia, the diagnosis is "personality change due to a general medical condition."

D. In Alzheimer's disease, the change in personality is usually an exaggeration of premorbid personality traits.

E. "Personality disorder not otherwise specified" is diagnosed rarely in elderly patients.

22.2   Personality disorder diagnosis in the elderly is subject to some specific clinical and epidemiological considerations. Which of the following is true?

A. The prevalence of personality disorders in the elderly population is approximately the same as in younger patients, about 10%.

B. The prevalence of personality disorders among elderly patients with another psychiatric condition is between 25% and 65%.

C. In the older population, the association between personality and anxiety disorders is the most often reported comorbidity.

D. Cluster B personality disorders do not improve with age.

E. The association between comorbid personality disorder and mood disorder is stronger for late-onset than for early-onset depression.

22.3   Vaillant's studies of the hierarchy of psychological defenses have been cited to explain personality function in old age. All of the following defense mechanisms are considered to be mature and thus adaptive *except*

A. Humor.
B. Altruism.
C. Repression.
D. Sublimation.
E. Suppression.

22.4 In the evaluation of personality disorders in the elderly patient, the physician can be assisted by several objective and semistructured instruments. Which of the following clinical assessment instruments is a semistructured interview rather than an ancillary self-report measure?

A. Millon Clinical Multiaxial Inventory—III (MCMI-III).
B. Personality Disorders Examination (PDE).
C. Personality Diagnostic Questionnaire (PDQ-IV).
D. Schedule for Nonadaptive and Adaptive Personality.
E. Wisconsin Personality Disorders Inventory.

22.5 Personality change due to degenerative frontal lobe disease is associated with difficulties in planning, conformity to social norms, experience of reward and punishment, and management of complex emotions. Clinically, these symptoms may bear strong resemblance to several DSM-IV-TR personality disorders. These specific behaviors may overlap with all of the following personality disorders *except*

A. Obsessive-compulsive.
B. Narcissistic.
C. Antisocial.
D. Borderline.
E. Paranoid.

Chapter 23

Agitation and Suspiciousness

Select the single best response for each question.

23.1 Which of the following is true regarding the psychotic disorder of late life referred to as late-life paraphrenia?

   A. It is the late-life recurrence of an earlier onset of schizophrenia in a patient who had been symptom-free for many years.
   B. According to Kraepelin's original description, most patients were male.
   C. Psychotic symptoms of the late-life episode typically include delusions, but hallucinations are not experienced.
   D. Patients have been reported to have simultaneous sensory deficits.
   E. Antipsychotics have been demonstrated to be effective for late-life delusional disorder.

23.2 The clinical evaluation of the suspicious and/or paranoid older patient requires consideration of specific concerns about psychotic disorders in older patients. Which of the following is true?

   A. Because of schizophrenic patients' tendency to isolate and have a shorter life expectancy, chronic paranoid schizophrenia is an infrequent cause of suspiciousness in elderly patients.
   B. Elderly schizophrenic patients are best managed with medication alone, rather than comprehensive treatment models.
   C. New-onset delusions in older patients are usually bizarre in nature.
   D. Antipsychotic medication should be used in all cases of sporadic agitation related to delusions.
   E. Agitation may follow family members' challenging of the patient's delusions.

23.3 When the physician evaluates the older patient with suspicious and/or paranoid complaints, which of the following is *not* recommended?

   A. Determine whether suspicious behavior is warranted; for example, consider the possibility of neglect or abuse.
   B. Challenge the delusion to verify that it is indeed fixed in the patient's mind.
   C. Obtain routine laboratory studies, including chemistry and complete blood count.
   D. Consider use of neuroimaging (e.g., CT or MRI of the head).
   E. Consider specialty referrals for vision and hearing examination and correction.

23.4 Agitation in dementia is a common clinical problem, for both the patient and the family. Which of the following is true regarding behavioral approaches to agitation in dementia?

A. Pharmacological approaches should precede nonpharmacological ones.
B. Patients with dementia are more likely to act out frustration with strangers than with family members because strangers are unfamiliar.
C. Agitation often correlates with other areas of impulsive behavior.
D. Because of their cognitive impairments, patients with dementia are usually nonresponsive to nonverbal behavior of caretakers.
E. Excessively calm, familiar surroundings and predictable routines unnecessarily understimulate the patient with dementia and thus should be avoided.

23.5 The pharmacological treatment of dementia with agitation is necessary in many cases. Which of the following is true?

A. Among antipsychotic agents, haloperidol is clearly superior at symptom control.
B. The atypical antipsychotic agents, though less likely to cause side effects, are limited in that there is no intramuscular formulation available.
C. When a patient has consistent episodes of behavioral agitation, medication should be used on an as-needed (PRN) basis.
D. The anticonvulsants carbamazepine and divalproex are also useful in dementia with agitation.
E. Selective serotonin reuptake inhibitor (SSRI) antidepressants should be used only in the context of clear mood symptoms.

23.6 Communication strategies in dementia may facilitate the patient's maintenance of behavioral control and avoidance of escalation into agitation. All of the following communication strategies are helpful *except*

A. Ensuring adequate vision and hearing correction.
B. Maintaining good eye contact and approaching the patient slowly.
C. Decreasing "clutter" in the sensory milieu (e.g., turning off noisy electronic equipment).
D. In assisting understanding, paraphrasing, rather than simply repeating, ideas that are not apparently understood.
E. Using specific names and references and avoiding pronouns and other nonspecific language devices.

Chapter 24

Psychopharmacology

Select the single best response for each question.

24.1 Psychopharmacological treatment of late-life psychiatric illness has significantly improved clinical function and quality of life for patients. However, systemic side effects from psychotropic medications are a vexing problem in this population. Many side effects are due to anticholinergic, antihistaminic, and antiadrenergic effects. All of the following clinical problems are referable to anticholinergic effects *except*

A. Constipation.
B. Urinary retention.
C. Sedation.
D. Delirium.
E. Cognitive dysfunction.

24.2 The selective serotonin reuptake inhibitors (SSRIs) have become the first-line agents in the treatment of mood disorders in older adults. Which of the following is true regarding the use of SSRIs in older patients?

A. Due to their pharmacokinetic profiles and low risk for drug-drug interactions, sertraline and fluoxetine are the preferred SSRIs.
B. Several controlled trials have demonstrated the effectiveness of SSRIs in anxiety disorders in elderly patients.
C. Despite not being technically "antipsychotic," SSRIs have been shown to be efficacious in treating delusions and hallucinations in dementia.
D. SSRIs may cause the syndrome of inappropriate secretion of antidiuretic hormone (SIADH) with hypernatremia, which may lead to delirium.
E. SSRIs are poorly tolerated in Parkinson's disease.

24.3 Other contemporary antidepressants may be clinically indicated in the older patient for various psychiatric symptoms. Which of the following is true?

A. Bupropion is contraindicated in seizure disorder patients, but it is recommended for poststroke depression.
B. Because it may energize a fatigued depressed patient, bupropion is the antidepressant of choice in psychotic depression.
C. Venlafaxine has different pharmacokinetic properties depending on the patient's age; thus, lower doses are typically effective for older patients.
D. The extended-release preparation of venlafaxine significantly reduces the risk for a withdrawal syndrome when treatment is interrupted or discontinued.
E. Mirtazapine inhibits 5-HT$_2$ and 5-HT$_3$ receptors, making it an attractive choice for elderly depressed patients with severe nausea.

24.4 Newer agents have largely supplanted the tricyclic antidepressants (TCAs). However, some TCAs may be useful for certain patients. The secondary, rather than tertiary, amine structures are associated with less side-effect burden. Which of the following TCAs is a secondary amine and thus likely to be more tolerable by older patients?

A. Amitriptyline.
B. Desipramine.
C. Imipramine.
D. Doxepin.
E. Clomipramine.

24.5 The atypical antipsychotic agents have been quickly integrated into geriatric psychiatric practice, as they are in general more tolerable than the older typical agents. Which of the following is true regarding this group of antipsychotic agents?

A. When used for drug-induced psychosis in Parkinson's disease, clozapine should be used at doses between 100 and 200 mg/day.
B. Olanzapine has been associated with elevated glucose and lipids, but only when there is simultaneous weight gain.
C. Because of risk of extrapyramidal symptoms in elderly patients, doses of risperidone should be limited to less than 1 mg/day.
D. Quetiapine does not show affinity for muscarinic receptors and is a viable alternative to clozapine for drug-induced psychosis in Parkinson's disease.
E. Ziprasidone's use in elderly patients is limited by its high degree of muscarinic receptor affinity and resultant risk of cognitive impairment.

24.6 Mood stabilizers may be useful in elderly patients, both for patients with long-established bipolar disorders and for behavioral acting-out in dementing illness. Which of the following is true?

A. Because of their greater safety profile in older patients, anticonvulsants are now prescribed much more commonly than lithium for elderly bipolar patients.
B. Older patients are subject to lithium toxicity at lower serum lithium levels than younger adults, with cognitive impairment reported at levels even lower than 1 mEq/L.
C. Although transient increases in liver-associated enzymes are seen in approximately 10% of patients treated with valproate, similar increases in serum ammonia are more rare.
D. Aging alone typically increases the half-life of valproate metabolism by a factor of 2 to 3.
E. Carbamazepine is a cytochrome P450 inhibitor and thus can inhibit its own metabolism, increasing serum levels.

24.7 Which of these cholinesterase inhibitors is notably affected by renal function and carries an FDA warning about dose titration?

A. Tacrine.
B. Donepezil.
C. Rivastigmine.
D. Galantamine.
E. Physostigmine.

Chapter 25

Electroconvulsive Therapy

Select the single best response for each question.

25.1 Electroconvulsive therapy (ECT) may be a useful intervention for several geriatric psychiatric conditions. Which of the following is true regarding ECT?

A. In recent years, studies have shown that fewer than 25% of patients receiving ECT are older than 65.
B. It has been conclusively shown that depression in elderly patients features more severe episodes that are more resistant to medication treatment.
C. ECT is effective in melancholic and psychotic depression, but not in nonmelancholic depression.
D. ECT may be effective for an acute manic episode.
E. ECT has a specifically beneficial effect on the "negative" or deficit symptoms of schizophrenia.

25.2 Which of the following is true regarding the use of ECT in elderly depressed patients?

A. Treatment response to ECT is lower in older patients.
B. Without maintenance treatment, less than half of successfully treated major depression cases will relapse in 6 months following ECT.
C. The relapse rate for depression following successful ECT treatment is the same whether or not the depressive episode leading to ECT was itself medication-resistant.
D. Randomized, controlled trials have demonstrated the benefit of maintenance ECT.
E. Maintenance pharmacotherapy is routinely recommended following a course of ECT unless prophylactic pharmacotherapy has previously failed.

25.3 While ECT is generally considered a second- or third-line treatment for a severe episode of depression or mania, there are certain instances where an urgent need for ECT may exist. This may be the case when the patient's condition is urgently life-threatening. All of the following circumstances would be considered life-threatening *except*

A. Extreme, constant suicidality.
B. Malnutrition because of poor oral intake.
C. Dehydration because of poor oral intake.
D. Psychosis.
E. Inability to comply with management of a critical additional medical problem.

25.4 Cognitive side effects following ECT may be quite distressing and may lead to treatment modification. Which of the following is true?

A. Anterograde amnesia usually resolves more slowly than retrograde amnesia following ECT.
B. Because of anterograde and retrograde amnesia, patients do not report an improvement in memory following ECT, despite improvement in mood.
C. While patients receiving lithium are more prone to cognitive side effects after ECT, preexisting cerebral disease is not a risk factor.
D. A larger number of ECT treatments and less time between treatments increase the risk of cognitive side effects.
E. Unilateral electrode placement increases the risk compared to bilateral placement.

25.5 Increased intracranial pressure at the time of ECT has led to extreme caution about applying ECT in patients with certain CNS illnesses. Despite this concern, the risk of CNS complications remains quite low. Which of the following conditions is *not* considered a space-occupying lesion in determining the advisability of ECT?

A. Normal-pressure hydrocephalus.
B. Subdural hematoma.
C. Intracranial arachnoid cyst.
D. Arteriovenous malformation.
E. CNS tumor.

25.6 At the time of ECT, certain psychoactive drugs should be temporarily discontinued to facilitate a successful treatment episode. All of the following psychotropic medications should be held at the time of ECT treatment *except*

A. Lithium.
B. Benzodiazepines.
C. Selective serotonin reuptake inhibitors (SSRIs).
D. Bupropion.
E. Clozapine.

25.7 The pre-ECT evaluation is critical in determining which patient receives ECT with the highest degree of safety. All of the following should be included in the pre-ECT evaluation in every case *except*

A. Full psychiatric history and examination.
B. Formal neuropsychological assessment of cognitive status.
C. Medical history and examination.
D. Dental history and examination for loose/missing teeth.
E. Anesthetic history and airway assessment.

C h a p t e r   2 6

Diet, Nutrition, and Exercise

Select the single best response for each question.

26.1   Assessment of nutritional status in older patients is facilitated by the use of objective measures. Numerous methods of nutritional status are available. Which of the following statements is true?

   A. Standard height and weight tables are reliable in elderly patients.
   B. Visceral protein stores are assessed by careful measurement of midarm circumference.
   C. The most widely accepted serum marker substances for protein stores are hemoglobin and ammonia.
   D. Water immersion is an accurate measure of body fat stores and is generally well tolerated by the patient.
   E. Although accuracy and precision are questioned, waist and hip circumference and skin-fold caliper measurements are effective clinical tools to assess nutritional status.

26.2   In parallel with protein and fat stores assessment, functional assessment of immune function is important in older patients. Which of the following is true?

   A. Skin tests for immune function assess beta-lymphocyte activity.
   B. Fungal antigens are injected subcutaneously.
   C. Antigens commonly used include *Candida* and *Trichophyton*.
   D. Since many healthy people are not reactive to these antigens, false positives are a consideration.
   E. Inadequate diet is not reflected in the total lymphocyte count unless the level is less than 1,000/mL.

26.3   Prescribed medications commonly used by elderly patients with chronic systemic conditions may have effects on vitamin and nutritional requirements. Which of the following is true?

   A. Trimethoprim and phenytoin increase the need for vitamins A and E and folate.
   B. Barbiturates and cholestyramine may deplete iron and B-complex vitamins, leading to need for supplementation.
   C. Neomycin and colchicine influence absorption of fat-soluble vitamins.
   D. Patients consuming a normal diet are commonly affected by medication-induced vitamin-deficiency states.
   E. Chronic atrophic gastritis has been associated with reduced absorption of nutrients, but not elevated absorption.

26.4 Dietary changes have been recommended as primary preventive therapy for many chronic conditions seen in elderly patients. Which of the following is true?

    A. An emphasis on fish and grains in the diet may stabilize, but not reverse, atherosclerotic lesions.

    B. Dietary factors are as significant in cancer risk as are environmental factors and smoking.

    C. The relation between obesity and pancreatic cancer has been linked to vascular disease, not insulin levels.

    D. Diets high in saturated fats have been conclusively linked to increased risk of breast, colon, and prostate cancer.

    E. A high-fiber diet has been associated with decreased risk of both diverticula and colon cancer.

26.5 Tertiary prevention refers to using nutritional modification to change the course of an established disease process. Which of the following is true?

    A. Osteoporosis is associated with calcium deficiency; fortunately, calcium supplements are benign, with few problematic side effects.

    B. In type 2 diabetes, the Western diet adversely affects the course of the illness but not its incidence.

    C. Sodium restriction to decrease intravascular volume is necessary in all edematous states, including congestive heart failure and renal failure.

    D. Elevated homocysteine levels increase risk for dementia; this risk can be modified by supplemental folate.

    E. Cruciferous vegetables (e.g., cauliflower and broccoli) in the diet decrease stroke risk, while other fruits and vegetables do not.

26.6 Exercise is an important component of overall well-being and can be neglected in the care of older patients. Which of the following is true?

    A. In diabetic patients, exercise will increase the need for insulin.

    B. The exercise tolerance test (ETT) should be obtained routinely in all community-based exercise programs.

    C. The ETT's greatest value is its accurate prediction of future exercise-related cardiac events.

    D. Obesity levels are primarily due to activity level, not diet.

    E. Maintaining exercise that produces a heart rate between 60% and 70% of maximal heart rate minimizes medical risks from exercise.

Chapter 27

Individual and Group Psychotherapy

Select the single best response for each question.

27.1   Psychotherapy may be a preferred model for certain geropsychiatric conditions. Which of the following is true regarding the general issue of psychotherapy for older patients?

   A. Because of the availability of Medicare, over 50% of older patients with psychiatric illnesses receive professional mental health care, unlike younger patients for whom insurance coverage is often problematic.
   B. Descriptive research regularly shows that older patients prefer psychopharmacological treatment to psychotherapy.
   C. Part of older patients' preference for psychopharmacological therapy is because few elders are concerned about "addiction" to antidepressants.
   D. Objective research confirms that "relationship factors" account for 80% of the variance in treatment outcomes with psychotherapy.
   E. The Luborsky meta-meta-analysis concluded that many psychotherapy models are equivalent in producing therapeutic gain.

27.2   When conducting psychotherapy with older patients, several factors specific to this age group should be taken into close account. All of the following are true *except*

   A. Older adults rarely respond to therapeutic interventions used with younger patients.
   B. Medical illnesses or medications may exacerbate psychiatric symptoms.
   C. The clinician must work against stereotypes about elderly patients.
   D. Older adults may not easily remember troubling earlier life events.
   E. Cognitive deficits may affect the progress of psychotherapy.

27.3   Cognitive-behavioral psychotherapy models may be considered for older patients. Which of the following is true?

   A. Behavioral activation and automatic thought modification are equally effective at preventing relapse, and there is a powerful synergistic effect when the techniques are combined.
   B. The Blumenthal et al. study (1999) showed that the medication plus exercise group improved significantly more than the exercise-only group.
   C. The Thompson et al. study (1987) showed cognitive and behavioral therapy to be superior to brief psychodynamic therapy in reducing depression symptoms.
   D. The studies by Thompson et al. (2001) and Reynolds et al. (1999) both concluded that combined medication and psychotherapy were optimal in the treatment of depression in older adults.
   E. A logistical limitation of social problem-solving therapy is that it is not adaptable to the primary care clinic.

27.4 Another useful model for psychotherapy for depressed older adults is interpersonal psychotherapy (IPT). This model is based on four components of interpersonal relationships that lead to and maintain depressive states. These four components include all of the following *except*

A. Grief.
B. Interpersonal disputes.
C. Role transitions.
D. Interpersonal deficits.
E. Intrapsychic or psychodynamic conflict.

27.5 Various psychotherapy models can be utilized for the management of anxiety disorders in older patients. Which of the following is true?

A. The most frequently used and well-substantiated psychotherapy model for geriatric anxiety symptoms is cognitive-behavioral therapy (CBT).
B. Behavioral therapy such as progressive muscle relaxation training is contraindicated for patients with cognitive impairment.
C. CBT appears to be the best-equipped psychotherapy model for generalized anxiety disorder (GAD) in older patients.
D. A major limitation of CBT for geriatric anxiety states is that it cannot be conducted in the primary care clinic.
E. Elderly patients with GAD infrequently exhibit simultaneous depressive symptoms.

27.6 Dementia is a common condition in geropsychiatry, and psychotherapy may be a valuable adjunctive treatment option in the comprehensive care of these patients. Which of the following is true?

A. Most empirical research on psychotherapy models for dementia is based on CBT.
B. Reality orientation therapy for dementia has been shown to improve mastery of activities of daily living in patients with dementia.
C. Validation therapy consists of empathic efforts to reinforce dementia patients' limited abilities to communicate.
D. Caregiver interventions should focus solely on behavior management of the patient with dementia and not on caregiver self-care.
E. Validation therapy is clearly more effective than general increased social support in accomplishing treatment gains.

Chapter 28

Working With the Family of the Older Adult

Select the single best response for each question.

28.1 Which of the following is true regarding care of elderly patients with dementia in the community?

A. Fifty percent of older patients with moderate or severe dementia live alone with some level of supervision.

B. Spousal caregiver strain from care for patients with dementia is associated with increased risk of premature death.

C. Anxiety symptoms are the most commonly reported psychiatric symptoms in caregivers of patients with dementia.

D. Dependent elders are much more likely to engage in manipulative behavior than to have legitimate unmet dependency needs.

E. Defensive denial of inevitable bad outcomes in dementia must be discouraged and avoided for caregivers to give appropriate dementia care.

28.2 In working with dementia patients and their families, psychiatrists are advised to attend to many parallel issues in both patients and family members. All of the following are true *except*

A. Psychiatrists should monitor the mental health of caregivers as well as patients.

B. Caregivers' self-neglect and patient neglect by caregivers are both important areas for surveillance.

C. Major precipitants of the decision to place a patient with dementia in an institution are both patient factors and caregiver factors.

D. While possibly problematic, affective, anxiety, and substance abuse disorders of caregivers do not themselves predict breakdown of family care models.

E. Disruptive psychiatric symptoms by the patient with dementia strongly predict institutional placement.

28.3 The conduct of office visits with dementia patients and family caregivers calls for the psychiatrist to make certain commonsense changes to clinical routine. Which of the following is true?

A. The psychiatrist should rigorously preserve patient confidentiality and not speak to family members unless the patient is present.

B. The patient should not be accompanied to the physician's office by more than one family member as this confuses the patient and leads to excessive boundary management challenges.

C. Older couples with long relationships often prefer to face medical challenges together rather than singly.

D. Psychiatrists should not encourage family members to remove weapons from the home of patients with dementia, as this is an invasion of privacy.

E. The psychiatrist should not encourage physical activity for the patient with dementia as the patient needs to preserve energy for cognitive tasks.

28.4   The psychiatrist caring for patients with dementia also needs to assess the family members of the patient. Which of the following is *not* true?

A. Older husbands who are caregivers are at increased risk of alcohol abuse.
B. Caregivers should be encouraged to pursue regular exercise.
C. The caregiver has a need for social stimulation while caring for a dependent elder.
D. Secondary family support should be assessed.
E. The psychiatrist should not directly address the caregiver's own health, as this is a matter for that person's own physician.

28.5   When handling diagnostic/prognostic communications and while recommending additional services to the family of patients with dementia, which of the following is true?

A. Some Asian American families regard use of formal supportive services as a moral failure.
B. Families rarely tolerate the demands of terminal care of an immobile and incontinent patient but can usually manage the disruptive sleep and behavior of moderate dementia.
C. Combined interventions, while appealing, have not been shown to decrease caregiver depression.
D. Health care decisions should not be made until the diagnosis of dementia is clear and there have been several months of follow-up to estimate rapidity of progression.
E. Families should be advised that judgment about financial matters is usually unimpaired in early dementia.

28.6   Driving is often a contentious issue in dementia. Which of the following is *not* true regarding driving by cognitively impaired patients?

A. Dementia leads to decreased judgment.
B. Increased reaction time is common in dementia.
C. Patients with dementia will respect the loss of their driver's license and cease to try to drive.
D. Mechanically disabling the car reduces the need to confront the patient with his or her lost skills.
E. Families should proactively arrange for alternative transportation to decrease the incentive for the patient to try to drive.

Chapter 29

Clinical Psychiatry in the Nursing Home

Select the single best response for each question.

29.1   Which of the following is true in the United States according to the 1995 National Nursing Home Survey (Gabrel and Jones 2000)?

   A. Between 9% and 10% of U.S. residents over the age of 65 resided in nursing homes.
   B. Compared to an earlier survey done in 1985, the percentage of older adults residing in nursing homes had increased by 0.5%.
   C. Between 1985 and 1995, the mean age of nursing home residents had increased by 2.9 years.
   D. Over 50% of women older than 85 lived in nursing homes.
   E. Among nursing home residents over 65, over 40% had vision and hearing impairments.

29.2   The prevalence of psychiatric disorders in nursing home residents has been the subject of several studies. Which of the following is *not* true?

   A. Interview-based studies have found prevalence rates of psychiatric illness in nursing home residents as high as 94%.
   B. The Rovner et al. study (1990) found that two-thirds of nursing home residents had dementia.
   C. The Medical Expenditures Panel Survey (MEPS) found a rate of depressive disorders in nursing home residents of 20%.
   D. The MEPS study was based on clinical interviews.
   E. Rovner et al. (1990) found a prevalence of psychiatric illness of 80% in new nursing home admissions.

29.3   Among psychiatric illnesses in nursing home residents, disorders of cognitive impairment are of great importance. Which of the following is true?

   A. Among dementia subtypes, Alzheimer's disease accounts for 75% of cases, with Lewy body dementia the second most common dementia.
   B. Delirium has been found in 20% of nursing home residents, primarily due to underlying dementia.
   C. Psychotic symptoms are seen in 25%–50% of dementia patients in nursing homes.
   D. Most psychiatric consultations in nursing homes are for psychotic episodes.
   E. Behavioral disturbance in dementia is solely due to cognitive impairment.

29.4 In addition to cognitive disorders, mood disorders are common psychiatric illnesses in nursing home residents. Which of the following is true?

A. Depressive disorders are the second most common psychiatric illness in nursing home residents.
B. The rate of mood disorders in nursing home residents in the United States is substantially higher than in other industrialized nations.
C. Depression in nursing home residents increases morbidity, but not mortality, rates.
D. Because of concurrent chronic medical illnesses, the DSM-IV-TR diagnostic criteria for mood disorders are not clinically valid in nursing home residents.
E. There is a subtype of depression in nursing home residents featuring low serum albumin, high levels of psychosocial disability, and prompt response to treatment with nortriptyline.

29.5 Intervention for psychiatric illnesses in nursing home residents is a major clinical focus of the geropsychiatrist. Which of the following is true?

A. A program of daytime physical activity and nursing interventions to promote nighttime sleep may decrease depression, but not agitation.
B. Outcome studies on psychotherapy models in nursing home residents are derived from illness-specific interventions.
C. Risperidone has been shown to have a beneficial effect on psychotic symptoms but not independent effects on agitation or aggression.
D. Risperidone has been repeatedly demonstrated to have beneficial long-term effects on psychosis in nursing home residents.
E. The majority of nursing home residents who are withdrawn from antipsychotic agents do not experience a reemergence of psychosis.

29.6 Several concerns noted in the 1970s and 1980s in the United States led to various legal and regulatory initiatives to improve the psychiatric care in nursing homes. Which of the following is true?

A. A 1977 survey in the United States revealed that 10% of nursing home residents were physically restrained.
B. Mechanical restraints independently decrease physical agitation.
C. Nursing home patients with nonpsychotic causes of agitation nonetheless require antipsychotic medications.
D. The 1986 Institute of Medicine report found that antipsychotic drugs were being overused in nursing homes.
E. The 1986 Institute of Medicine report found that antidepressant drugs were being overused in nursing homes.

29.7 In the United States, federal regulation has led to modified practices in nursing homes. Which of the following is true?

A. An initial first-stage screening looking for mental disorders in nursing home admissions specifically includes dementia.
B. The second-stage assessment requires a psychiatric evaluation.
C. Patients with dementia are required to have both a psychiatric and a neurological evaluation.
D. The Minimum Data Set (MDS) must be administered only once to a nursing home resident.
E. Resident Assessment Protocols (RAPs) are solely for monitoring of the use of psychotropic medication.

29.8 Concern had been raised about the use of "unnecessary drugs" in psychiatrically ill nursing home patients. All of the following constitute an "unnecessary drug" use *except*

A. Drug used at an excessive dose.
B. Drug used for excessive duration.
C. Drug used with inadequate monitoring.
D. Drug used despite adverse consequences.
E. Drug used for other than FDA-approved indications ("off-label").

Chapter 30

The Continuum of Care: Movement Toward the Community

Select the single best response for each question.

30.1   The trends toward community-based care rather than institutionally based care have been subject to many demographic and epidemiological variables as well as policy and programmatic considerations. Which of the following is true?

    A.   Primarily due to the burgeoning of the elderly population living longer with chronic illness, disability in the U.S. population has been increasing at the rate of 2% per year for the past several decades.

    B.   Between 1983 and 2003, the occupancy rate at available nursing homes has increased steadily.

    C.   Medicare devotes a large percentage of its resources to long-term care.

    D.   Community-based care for chronically impaired adults is lower cost than institutional care.

    E.   Recent initiatives for long-term care models come not from federal initiatives but from a series of organizations such as professional and community organizations.

30.2   The set of specific judgments by individuals that they can perform competently and capably in specific situations is referred to as

    A.   Self-esteem.
    B.   Self-efficacy.
    C.   Collective efficacy.
    D.   Actualization.
    E.   Ego integrity.

30.3   The movement toward hospice care for terminally ill patients has been a major innovation in community-based care. Which of the following is *not* true regarding hospice care?

    A.   In both England and the United States, hospice emphasizes home care rather than institutional care.

    B.   A major emphasis in hospice care is adequacy of pain management.

    C.   Hospice care in the United States is covered by Medicare.

    D.   Hospice care at end of life reduces costs.

    E.   Hospice care is an appropriate model for both cancer and AIDS patients.

30.4 Assisted living models may be a useful alternative care plan for many elderly patients with support needs. Which of the following is true?

A. In the United States, older patients are more likely to be in substandard housing than adults of all other age groups.
B. The majority of older adults in the United States live alone.
C. Assisted living housing includes a private, self-contained personal living space.
D. Responsibility for care is solely limited to patients and families.
E. Assisted living is a low-cost option for frail elders, with few economic barriers to access to this model.

30.5 An easily neglected problem is housing and support for chronic mentally ill patients who have grown old. Which of the following is true?

A. The broadening of mental health programs in the 1970s specifically addressed the mental health needs of older patients.
B. Mental health "carve-outs" control costs solely by limiting psychiatric hospital utilization.
C. In the United States, the Older Americans Act specifically addresses the mental health needs of the elderly.
D. In the United States, federal funding through the Administration on Aging mandates specific mental health program funding at the community level.
E. Because of the existence of clear federal policies on mental health care of older patients, this issue is not considered a state or local responsibility.

30.6 The Robert Wood Johnson Foundation's Community Partnership for Older Adults program was established in 2001 to enhance community care models. Which of the following is *not* true regarding this initiative?

A. Blends collaborative community partnerships and knowledgeable consumers.
B. Mobilizes community to create awareness of contributions and needs of older citizens.
C. Educates consumers to become more informed.
D. Promotes better quality of care and quality of life within existing and new programs.
E. Leverages solely private financial resources to meet identified community needs.

Chapter 31

Legal, Ethical, and Policy Issues

Select the single best response for each question.

31.1 Medicare provides funding for a great deal of medical and mental health care to older patients in the United States. Which of the following is true regarding this program and mental health care?

A. Psychotropic medication management is subject to a 50% copayment from the patient.

B. To enhance the use of lower-cost service models, Medicare payment policies discourage acute inpatient psychiatric hospitals while encouraging outpatient psychiatric care.

C. There is a 190-day lifetime limit for inpatient psychiatric care, which pertains to both freestanding and general hospital-based psychiatric units.

D. Despite the benefits available in Medicare, only 6%–8% of older adults receive outpatient mental health services.

E. Medicare Part C plans with managed care programs have become the choice of 50% of older patients.

31.2 Which of the following is *not* true regarding federal regulation of nursing homes in the United States?

A. Regulatory concern in the 1980s focused on the inappropriate use of chemical restraints.

B. Regulatory concern in the 1980s focused on the inappropriate use of physical restraints.

C. In the 1980s, there was concern that antidepressants were being prescribed excessively in nursing homes.

D. The Omnibus Budget Reconciliation Act of 1987 contained the Nursing Home Reform Act; this act addressed mental health care issues in nursing homes.

E. Nursing home applicants must now have a preadmission assessment to establish psychiatric needs and appropriate placement.

31.3 The Health Care Financing Administration (HCFA) in 1999 introduced 24 quality indicators for nursing homes. Quality indicators pertinent to geriatric psychiatry include all of the following *except*

A. Behavior problems.

B. Emotional problems.

C. Cognitive patterns.

D. Psychotropic drug use.

E. Percentage of patients receiving psychiatric consultation.

31.4   Ethical issues at the end of life are an important consideration in the care of the older patient. Which of the following is *not* included in the Joint Commission on Accreditation of Healthcare Organizations core principles for end-of-life care?

A. Respect dignity of patient and caregivers.
B. Encompass alleviation of pain and other physical symptoms.
C. Assess and manage psychosocial problems.
D. Provide access to palliative and/or hospice care.
E. Limit access to potentially harmful nonvalidated treatments, such as alternative and nontraditional treatments.

31.5   Which of the following is true regarding advance directives?

A. Patients receiving care funded by Medicare or Medicaid are required to execute advance directives.
B. A power of attorney for health care requires notarization in all 50 U.S. states.
C. "Durable power of attorney" is synonymous with "legal guardianship."
D. A living will confers a wider scope of decision making than a power of attorney for health care.
E. Compliance with advance directives by medical institutions remains poor.

31.6   Which of the following is true regarding legal competency for decision making?

A. Competency can be determined by the decision of any psychiatrist.
B. Competency can be determined by the decision of a psychiatrist, only if he or she is board-certified.
C. Competency requires a court decision, not a medical one.
D. Making a will and executing a power of attorney require the same level of competency.
E. The court may request a written report but may not compel the physician to personally testify in competency cases.

Chapter 32

The Past and Future of Geriatric Psychiatry

Select the single best response for each question.

32.1 Which is true regarding the roles of the National Institute on Aging (NIA), the National Institute of Mental Health (NIMH), Medicare, and other sponsoring agencies in geriatric psychiatry?

    A. The NIA is the office of responsibility for research into psychiatric illnesses affecting the elderly population, for example, major depression.

    B. The NIMH leads efforts on Alzheimer's disease research.

    C. The NIMH is responsible for direct funding support for over 50% of geriatric psychiatric fellowships.

    D. The Department of Veterans Affairs (VA) supports the most comprehensive system of care for mentally ill older adults in the United States.

    E. Medicare's capitation payments system using diagnosis-related groups (DRGs) is applied to inpatient psychiatric care.

32.2 Geriatric psychiatrists may practice preventive psychiatry in many instances. Which of the following interventions would be a primary prevention effort?

    A. Provision of adequate social and logistical support to decrease loneliness and despair, preventing the onset of major psychiatric illness.

    B. Early diagnosis of major depression and provision of supportive psychotherapy.

    C. Early diagnosis of major depression and provision of supportive psychotherapy plus pharmacotherapy.

    D. Early diagnosis of major depression and provision of pharmacotherapy.

    E. Rehabilitation of patients with dementia who are managed in a long-term care facility.

32.3 The concept of "successful aging" is associated with the concept of "wisdom" as articulated by Baltes (1993). Which of the following is *not* included under the components of wisdom as described by Baltes?

    A. Factual knowledge.

    B. Procedural knowledge.

    C. Life-span contextualization.

    D. Value absolutism.

    E. Acceptance of uncertainty.

32.4 Which is true regarding the subspecialty board certification in geriatric psychiatry in the United States?

    A. The first examination was given in 1981.

    B. Applicants must now complete a 1-year fellowship in geriatric psychiatry to take the examination.

    C. Certifications are for 5 years.

    D. Recertifying examinations are closed-book format.

    E. The added credential is officially called "Added Qualifications in Geriatric Psychiatry."

Chapter 1

The Myth, History, and Science of Aging

Select the single best response for each question.

1.1   Hayflick is noted as having determined that

A. Cells continue to divide at a fairly even rate throughout life.
B. Cells double at a rate inversely proportional to age.
C. Frozen cells thawed years later now divide at a rejuvenated rate; memory of the number of prior doublings is "forgotten."
D. Death of a cell line is usually due to faulty laboratory techniques.
E. The only human cells that may be immortal are mixoploid cells, such as HeLa cells.

The correct response is option B.

Several investigators have replicated the work of Hayflick, finding that the number of population doublings of cultured human cells is inversely proportional to donor age.

It appears that the only human cells that may be immortal are transformed or abnormal mixoploid cells such as the HeLa cells, which were originally taken from cancerous cervical tissue and grown in culture by George O. Gey in 1950. The death of a cell line was usually attributed to failure to use proper laboratory methods. It was subsequently shown that freezing viable normal human cells at subzero temperatures does not alter the memory in the cells for the number of doublings that had previously occurred. **(p. 4)**

1.2   Aging is usually considered

A. Necessarily confined to the latter years of life.
B. To result in a decline in efficiency of function, reduce homeostasis, and terminate in death.
C. To not particularly involve changes in striated musculature.
D. To result in diminished capacity for storage of drugs.
E. To result in declines of tyrosine hydroxylase, cholinesterase, and monoamine oxidase.

MAO ↑ with age

The correct response is option B.

Aging designates those physical changes that develop in adulthood, result in a decline in efficiency of function, reduce homeostasis, and terminate in death.

Drugs are metabolized in elderly people differently than the way they are metabolized in younger adults. Striated musculature diminishes by about one-half by approximately age 80 years. As these muscle cells disappear, they are replaced by fat cells and fibrous connective tissue. Hence, the body achieves increased storage capacities for certain drugs that are stored in fat cells. Aging results in a decline of neurotransmitters such as dopamine, norepinephrine, serotonin, tyrosine hydroxylase, and cholinesterase. The activity of monoamine oxidase increases with age. **(pp. 6–7)**

1.3   Major advantages of aging include all of the following *except*

A. The aged are much better citizens and interested in public issues and political affairs.
B. Older workers are stable but have more absenteeism.
C. In general, older persons are much less likely to be the victims of crime than people of other age groups.
D. Older persons maintain voluntary participation in community organizations, churches, and recreational groups.
E. Social Security and other pension systems have improved the economic status of older persons.

The correct response is option B.

Older workers are stable and dependable and have less absenteeism.

The aged are much better citizens and are interested and active in public issues and political affairs. They make an enormous contribution to society by maintaining voluntary participation in community organizations, churches, and recreational groups. Although older persons are equally exposed to crimes of certain types, they are much less likely to be the victims of crime in general than are people in other age groups. Although some of the apparent advantages of aged individuals are under constant pressure, it is obvious that Social Security and other pension systems have improved their economic status, as have lower taxes and other economic benefits such as reduced rates in many hotels, motels, and recreational facilities. **(p. 6)**

1.4   Timing of age-related change is thought to involve all of the following *except*

A. Cell loss within clusters of the hypothalamus.
B. Telomere shortening and cellular senescence.
C. Oxygen free radicals.
D. Decrease in the immune competence and alterations in the regulation of the immune system.
E. Loss of glycated forms of human collagen in tendon and skin with age.

The correct response is option E.

The aging chain alters the characteristics of connective tissue. Glycated forms of human collagen do accumulate with age in tendon and skin.

Cell loss, an event that is common in late life, occurs within clusters of cells in the hypothalamus, which causes other endocrine changes. Telomere shortening and cellular senescence have been well established in the laboratory. The oxygen free radical, superoxide, is an important agent of oxygen toxicity and the aging process. Considerable evidence has accumulated that a decrease in the immune competence and alterations in the regulation of the immune system are associated with aging. **(pp. 8–9)**

1.5   The differential in life expectancy between men and women is thought to involve all of the following *except*

A. Death rates by accidents and other violent causes are higher for men than for women.
B. Ischemic heart disease is consistently higher for men than for women.
C. There is greater incidence of cigarette smoking among men.
D. Malignancies are less frequent among males than among females over most of the life span.
E. There are differences in smoking habits between men and women.

The correct response is option D.

Malignancies are more frequent among males than among females over most of the life span.

Death rates by accidents and other violent causes are much higher for men than for women. Ischemic heart disease has been consistently higher for men than for women in almost all available international and historical data. In contemporary industrial societies, the single most important cause of higher mortality for males has been a greater incidence of cigarette smoking among men. Men smoke more cigarettes per day and inhale more deeply than do women. **(pp. 10–11)**

Chapter 2

Demography and Epidemiology of Psychiatric Disorders in Late Life

Select the single best response for each question.

2.1   The "old-old" populace (older than age 85) is projected to reach what number of persons by the year 2050?

A. 10 million.
B. 12 million.
C. 20 million.
D. 25 million.
E. 27 million.

The correct response is option C.

The oldest old among us are projected to reach 20 million by the year 2050 and to make up 5% of the United States population at that time. **(p. 17)**

2.2   The geriatric population is expected to increase to how many by the year 2030?

A. 30 million.
B. 40 million.
C. 50 million.
D. 60 million.
E. 70 million.

The correct response is option E.

The size of the elderly population in the United States is expected to dramatically increase in the next decades, reaching 70 million by the year 2030. **(p. 17)**

2.3   Case identification in geriatrics is particularly germane because

A. Distinction between a case and a noncase is easily established.
B. Epidemiologists cannot assist the clinician in identifying meaningful clusters of symptoms.
C. Many of the symptoms and signs of a psychiatric disorder in late life may be ubiquitous with the aging process.
D. Clinicians particularly favor case identification based on severity of functional impediment.
E. Most older adults ideally fit the psychiatric diagnosis they receive.

The correct response is option C.

Many of the symptoms and signs of a psychiatric disorder in late life may be ubiquitous with the aging process, thus blurring the distinction between cases and noncases.

The absolute distinction between a case and a noncase—that is, persons requiring psychiatric attention versus those who do not require such care—is not easily established. Epidemiologists can assist the clinician in identifying meaningful clusters of symptoms and significant degrees of symptom severity. Some authors define a case on the basis of severity of physical, psychological, and social impairment secondary to the symptoms. This approach to case identification is less popular among clinicians, who are more inclined to "treat a disease" than to "improve function." Most older adults do not ideally fit the psychiatric diagnosis that they receive. **(p. 18)**

2.4   The NIMH ECA program (1984) established the two most prevalent disorders of the elderly as

   A. Depressive and anxiety disorders.
   B. Depressive and cognitive disorders.
   C. Depressive and psychotic disorders.
   D. Anxiety and cognitive disorders.
   E. Anxiety and psychotic disorders.

The correct response is option D.

According to the NIMH ECA program (Regier et al. 1984), the two most prevalent disorders in people age 65 or older were an anxiety disorder (5.5%) and severe cognitive impairment (4.9%) (Regier et al. 1988). **(p. 20)**

2.5   The most frequently reported psychiatric symptom(s) of the elderly is (are)

   A. Depression.
   B. Fatigue.
   C. Problems with sleep.
   D. Anxiety related.
   E. C and D.

The correct response is option E.

The most frequently reported symptoms are problems with sleep and symptoms of anxiety. **(p. 21)**

2.6   Suicide in the elderly

   A. Is highest in the 65–74 sector.
   B. Is highest in the 78–84 sector.
   C. Is inversely correlated with age.
   D. Is most pronounced in white men older than 70.
   E. Has demonstrated a cohort effect of an increased rate with more modern manufacture of domestic gas.

The correct response is option D.

The highest suicide rates are found in white males older than 70.

Suicide rates have been positively correlated with age. The rate of gas poisoning has dramatically decreased with the conversion of domestic gas to methane. **(p. 27)**

2.7   Major depression has *not* been associated with

   A. Having functional limitation.
   B. External locus of control.
   C. Poorer self-perceived health.
   D. Perceived loneliness.
   E. Being unmarried.

The correct response is option B.

In the Longitudinal Aging Study Amsterdam (LASA; Beekman et al. 1995), major depression was associated with being unmarried; having functional limitation, perceived loneliness, internal locus of control, and poorer self-perceived health; and not receiving instrumental social support. **(p. 31)**

References

Beekman ATF, Deeg DJH, van Tilberg T, et al: Major and minor depression in later life: a study of prevalence and risk factors. J Affect Disord 36:65–75, 1995

Regier DA, Myers JK, Kramer M, et al: The NIMH Epidemiologic Catchment Area Program: historical context, major objectives and study population characteristics. Arch Gen Psychiatry 41:934–941, 1984

Regier DA, Boyd JH, Burke JD, et al: One-month prevalence of mental disorders in the United States. Arch Gen Psychiatry 45:977–986, 1988

Chapter 3

Physiological and Clinical Considerations of Geriatric Patient Care

Select the single best response for each question.

3.1   Falls in the elderly

    A. Are frequently multifactorial.
    B. Involve one-third of all community-dwelling elderly every year.
    C. Predict considerable morbidity.
    D. Promote risk for decline in instrumental activities of daily living.
    E. All of the above.

The correct response is option E.

Falls are generally multifactorial and are caused by intrinsic factors, situational factors, extrinsic factors, and medications. Half of all nursing home residents and one-third of all community-dwelling elderly have a fall every year. These falls produce notable morbidity. Those who fall frequently are at risk for a decline in their instrumental activities of daily living. **(p. 46)**

3.2   Urinary incontinence in the elderly is

    A. Most frequently stress incontinence in men.
    B. Most frequently overflow incontinence.
    C. Most frequently urge incontinence.
    D. Seen in up to one-half of community-residing elderly.
    E. None of the above.

The correct response is option C.

Half of all nursing home residents and up to one-third of persons older than 65 residing in the community carry the diagnosis of urinary continence.

Urge incontinence is the form of incontinence that has the highest prevalence in older patients. Stress incontinence is a frequent form of incontinence among elderly women, ranking second. Overflow incontinence is the second most prevalent type of incontinence in elderly men; often, it is produced by bladder outlet obstruction resulting from urethral strictures, benign prostatic hypertrophy, and prostate cancer. **(p. 47)**

3.3   The musculoskeletal system is affected in which of the following ways?

    A. Decrease in skeletal muscle mass.
    B. Increase in number of type II fibers.
    C. Age-associated changes in muscle mass and strength may be modified by exercise.
    D. A and B.
    E. A and C.

The correct response is option E.

In the fourth decade, both muscle mass and strength begin to decrease, and exercise may modify these age-associated changes.
     The number of type II fast-twitch fibers decreases in the elderly. **(pp. 42–43)**

3.4   Considerations in geriatric prescription should include all of the following *except*

    A. Volume of distribution.
    B. Absorption.
    C. Renal clearance.
    D. Oxidative metabolism in the cytochrome P450 system.
    E. Change in elimination half-life.

The correct response is option B.

Age has no significant effect on absorption, although acid secretion, gastrointestinal perfusion, and membrane transport all may decrease and thereby lower absorption. Gastrointestinal transit time is prolonged and increases absorption, and thus no net change occurs.
     The volume of distribution is significantly affected by the changes in body mass and total body water that occur with aging. With age, renal mass and renal blood flow are decreased, resulting in a decline in glomerular filtration rate and creatinine clearance. This decrease in clearance can alter the rate at which drugs are excreted, and dosages must be appropriately adjusted. Oxidative metabolism in the cytochrome P450 system is slower, thereby affecting elimination, but conjugation is not. The elimination half-life—the time required for the drug concentration to decrease by half—of certain drugs increases in the elderly and may be affected by the relation between volume of distribution or clearance; this may require adjustment of the drug dosing interval. **(p. 44)**

3.5   All of the following are true of the aging nervous system *except*

    A. Significant neuronal loss occurs in the locus coeruleus.
    B. Aging neuronal synapses may be decreased in the substantia nigra.
    C. Aging neuronal synapse size may be decreased in the substantia nigra.
    D. Aging neuronal synapse size may be increased.
    E. Protein and myelin content of the brain decreases.

The correct response is option C.

Aging neurons maintain the ability to make new synapses; the number of synapses may decrease, but their size may increase.
     Significant neuronal loss occurs in the locus coeruleus and the substantia nigra, and Purkinje's cells decrease in the cerebellum. The protein and myelin content of the brain decreases, and the brain becomes smaller and lighter. **(pp. 38–39)**

3.6   Which of the following is true of cognition in normal aging?

   A. Crystallized intelligence changes with age.
   B. Fluid intelligence begins to improve in the middle of the sixth decade and thereafter.
   C. Practical intelligence may be stable or even improve with age.
   D. Aging adults do not lose the ability to sustain attention over long periods.
   E. Short-term memory is affected.

   The correct response is option C.

   Practical intelligence, which tracks procedural skills, may be stable or even improve with age.
      Crystallized intelligence, an indication of accumulated knowledge or experience, does not change with age, but fluid intelligence, or novel problem-solving ability, begins to decline in the middle of the sixth decade and accelerates thereafter. Aging adults may lose their ability to sustain attention over long periods. Short-term, or working, memory is unaffected, but there may be problems in accessing data from long-term memory. **(p. 38)**

3.7   Ocular changes include which of the following?

   A. Weakening of the ciliary muscle.
   B. Photooxidation leading to yellowing of the lens.
   C. Decline in ability to view objects at rest.
   D. A and B.
   E. A, B, and C.

   The correct response is option E.

   The weakening of the ciliary muscle, combined with the loss of elasticity in the lens, results in presbyopia. Photooxidation leads to yellowing of the lens. The elderly also show a decline in their ability to view objects at rest (static acuity) and in motion (dynamic acuity). **(p. 39)**

3.8   Vascular changes of the elderly consist of all of the following *except*

   A. Elevated sympathetic nervous activity with increased level of circulating norepinephrine.
   B. Cardiac and vascular surface cell receptors less sensitive to norepinephrine.
   C. Beta-adrenergic response of the heart during exercise is exaggerated.
   D. A lower maximum heart rate.
   E. Less cardiac emptying.

   The correct response is option C.

   The beta-adrenergic response of the heart during exercise is attenuated; a lower maximum heart rate and decreased force of contraction are the result.
      Sympathetic nervous activity rises in the elderly patient, as evidenced by higher circulating levels of norepinephrine. Norepinephrine fills cardiac and vascular surface cell receptors, making them less sensitive. The older heart dilates during exercise to increase end-diastolic volume and maintain stroke volume, but cardiac output nonetheless declines with age. Because the heart stiffens, it empties less completely. **(p. 39)**

3.9   Gastrointestinal system changes of the elderly include

    A. Fewer myenteric ganglion cells.
    B. Diminished acid and pepsin production by the stomach.
    C. Diminished function of liver, gallbladder, and pancreas.
    D. Diminished ability of liver to manufacture binding proteins.
    E. Diminished liver transaminases and alkaline phosphatase.

The correct response is option A.

There are fewer myenteric ganglion cells, which affects the coordination of swallowing and may predispose some elderly patients to aspiration.

    The production of acid and pepsin by the stomach is mostly preserved. The liver, gallbladder, and pancreas continue to function well in the elderly patient. The liver's ability to manufacture binding proteins and metabolize drugs is stable, although considerable variability can be found between individuals. Liver transaminases and alkaline phosphatase remain unchanged. **(p. 40)**

3.10   Hormone levels are affected in all of the following ways *except*

    A. Decrease in growth hormone.
    B. Decrease in dehydroepiandrosterone.
    C. Decrease in cortisol.
    D. Increase in parathyroid hormone levels.
    E. Increase in sex-hormone binding globulin levels.

The correct response is option C.

Cortisol levels remain the same in the elderly because of a decrease in the cortisol metabolic clearance rate.

    Growth hormone (GH) declines because of both a decrease in growth hormone releasing hormone secretion and an increase in somatostatin. Both dehydroepiandrosterone (DHEA) and dehydroepiandrosterone sulfate (DHEA-S) decrease significantly in the elderly. Parathyroid hormone (PTH) levels are higher in the elderly because of increased secretion and decreased renal clearance. An increase in sex-hormone binding globulin levels limits the amount of free testosterone available. **(pp. 41–42)**

C h a p t e r   4

Neuroanatomy, Neurophysiology, and Neuropathology of Aging

Select the single best response for each question.

4.1   The limbic system

    A. Is involved in complex behaviors including the elaboration and expression of emotion.

    B. Is involved in learning and memory.

    C. Does not include the amygdala.

    D. A and B.

    E. A and C.

The correct response is option D.

The limbic system is involved in more complex behaviors, including the elaboration and expression of emotions, as well as learning and memory.

    The limbic structures include the amygdaloid complex, hippocampal formation, and cingulate gyrus. **(p. 64)**

4.2   EEG recordings of normal aging would not be expected to show

    A. Small increase in beta frequency.

    B. Small increase in theta frequency.

    C. Small increase in alpha frequency.

    D. No significant increase in delta frequency.

    E. Dominance of frequencies in the alpha range.

The correct response is option C.

A small decline in the mean alpha frequency may be seen beginning in the fifth decade.

    A small increase in beta frequency activity often correlates with age. Small increases in theta activity are frequently seen in healthy aged subjects but also may be associated with the subclinical onset of cerebrovascular disease. Normal aging is generally not associated with significant increases in delta activity. The EEG of a healthy awake adult is dominated by frequencies in the alpha range. **(p. 66)**

4.3   EEG changes with dementia include

   A. Decrease in delta and theta activity.
   B. Decreased coherence.
   C. Increase in beta activity.
   D. Increase in dominant alpha frequency.
   E. Change most frequently seen in the high-frequency band.

   The correct response is option B.

   Several studies have shown decreased coherence in dementia, which may reflect the loss of long corticocortical connections.
       The most characteristic EEG findings associated with dementia are an increase in low-frequency (delta and theta) activity, along with a decrease in high-frequency beta activity and slowing of the dominant alpha frequencies. The change in low-frequency band is best able to distinguish subjects with dementia from control subjects. **(p. 66)**

4.4   EEG findings in delirium would include

   A. Slowing.
   B. Quantitative EEG signal correlated with severity and duration of delirium.
   C. The finding that slowing cannot be meaningfully used in a patient with concomitant dementia.
   D. A and C.
   E. A and B.

   The correct response is option E.

   The EEG is a standard tool in the evaluation of delirium because EEG slowing is an almost universal finding in delirium. The quantitative EEG signal correlates with the severity and duration of the delirium.
       The degree of slowing reflects the severity of the delirium even in the context of preexisting dementia and therefore may be of particular use in detecting delirium as a complication of dementia. **(p. 66)**

4.5   Regarding seizures in the elderly, which of the following is true?

   A. Incidence is quite low.
   B. Approximately half are related to either strokes or tumors.
   C. Seizures rarely become recurrent.
   D. These patients would not be expected to demonstrate a normal EEG.
   E. Alzheimer's disease is rarely a risk factor.

   The correct response is option B.

   The incidence of seizures in the elderly is quite high and may account for up to one-quarter of new epilepsy cases. Approximately half of these seizures are related to either strokes or tumors, whereas up to a quarter have unknown causes; as many as 80% become recurrent.
       A high percentage of persons with seizures may have normal EEG findings. Alzheimer's dementia is a risk factor for refractory seizures in the elderly. **(p. 67)**

4.6   The P3 evoked potential wave

A. Is thought to reflect processes related to attention and immediate memory.
B. Increases in latency with age in normal subjects.
C. Increases in latency only in patients with dementia.
D. Is distinguishable between subtypes of cortical dementias.
E. A and B.

The correct response is option E.

The P3 wave is thought to reflect neural processes underlying attention and immediate memory and has been shown to increase in latency with age in normal subjects with little age-related change in other components of the evoked waveform.

The P3 latency is increased with normal aging and increases further in most patients with dementia. Studies of the P3 latency have not been able to distinguish between subtypes of cortical dementias. **(p. 67)**

4.7   Within normal aging

A. Approximately 30%–50% of elders show no evidence of cortical atrophy, cell loss, senile neuritic plaques, or neurofibrillary tangles.
B. Neuritic plaques or neurofibrillary tangles are not observed.
C. Distributional frequency of neuritic plaques consistently correlates with cognitive function.
D. Neurofibrillary tangle frequency and distribution do not predict cognitive function.
E. None of the above.

The correct response is option A.

Approximately 30%–50% of normally aged individuals show no evidence of cortical atrophy, no evidence of cell loss, no evidence of senile neuritic plaques, and no evidence of neurofibrillary tangles.

Both senile neuritic plaques and neurofibrillary tangles can be observed in normally aged individuals. The distribution and frequency of mature neuritic plaques do not consistently correlate with cognitive function. In contrast to this lack of correlation between neuritic plaques and cognition, neurofibrillary tangle frequency and distribution do predict cognitive status. **(p. 69)**

4.8   Alzheimer's disease is associated with which of the following?

A. Hirano bodies.
B. Granulovacuolar degeneration.
C. Asymmetrical atrophy and brain weight loss.
D. A and B.
E. A and C.

The correct response is option D.

Extracellular eosinophilic rods composed of actin filaments, known as Hirano bodies, are most commonly seen surrounding pyramidal neurons in the hippocampal formation. The frequency of Hirano bodies increases with age and with the severity of neurofibrillary change. Other pathology seen in Alzheimer's disease includes granulovacuolar degeneration, which was first described in 1911. Granulovacuoles occur within large pyramidal neurons of the hippocampal formation and amygdala.

The bilaterally symmetrical atrophy associated with Alzheimer's disease results in a 200- to 500-g weight loss. **(pp. 72–73)**

4.9   Dementia with Lewy bodies includes all of the following neuropathological correlates *except*

    A. Neurofibrillary tangles.
    B. Neuritic plaques.
    C. More Lewy bodies in the substantia nigra than in idiopathic Parkinson's disease.
    D. Alpha-synuclein expressed in Lewy bodies.
    E. Weight of the brain typically less than the weight of the brain of the patient with Alzheimer's disease.

The correct response is option E.

Generally, the weight of the brain of the patient with dementia with Lewy bodies is greater than the weight of the brain of the patient with Alzheimer's disease and may closely approximate normal.

Diffuse and neuritic plaques may be frequent, but neurofibrillary change is generally less intense than in "pure" Alzheimer's disease. The frequency of Lewy bodies in the substantia nigra of patients with dementia with Lewy bodies may be greater than in patients dying of idiopathic Parkinson's disease. Alpha-synuclein is a protein that has been found to be mutated in rare families with early-onset familial Parkinson's disease. **(pp. 73–74)**

Chapter 5

Chemical Messengers

Select the single best response for each question.

5.1   Cholinergic neurons have been shown

   A. To be major targets of degeneration in Alzheimer's disease.
   B. To be innervated by hypertrophied galanin terminals in Alzheimer's disease.
   C. To have large increases in the activity and number of high-affinity choline uptake transporter sites in Alzheimer's disease.
   D. A, B, and C.
   E. A and C.

The correct response is option D.

The cholinergic neurons have been shown to be one of the major targets of degeneration in Alzheimer's disease. The nucleus basalis acetylcholine (ACh) neurons are often found to contain the neuropeptide galanin, and the galanin terminals that innervate the ACh neurons in this region become hypertrophied in persons with Alzheimer's disease. Large increases (400%) in the activity and the number of high-affinity choline uptake transporter sites were observed in cortical tissue from patients with Alzheimer's disease compared with control subjects without dementia and those with dementia from a cause other than Alzheimer's disease. **(pp. 86–87)**

5.2   Changes of aging that occur in dopamine and dopamine receptors include

   A. Decreased numbers of D_2 receptors in the striatum with increasing age correlated with decreased cognitive function.
   B. Decreased dopamine transporter in caudate/putamen in oldest subjects.
   C. Correlation with decreased glucose metabolism of the frontal, temporal, and cingulate cortices.
   D. A, B, and C.
   E. None of the above.

The correct response is option D.

Decreased numbers of D_2 receptors in the striatum with increasing age have been correlated with decreasing cognitive function. The dopamine transporter declines slowly over the entire course of aging, not just at the end stages of life. A loss of dopamine D_2 receptor binding of $[^{11}C]$raclopride in the frontal, temporal, and cingulate cortices was significantly correlated with age-related decline in neuronal glucose metabolism in these regions. **(pp. 90–92)**

5.3   Serotonergic neurons

   A. Do not show alterations of tryptophan hydroxylase with increasing age.
   B. Show a 10% increase per decade in binding of 5-HT_{1A}.
   C. Show a 17% increase per decade of 5-HT_{2A} receptors.
   D. Increase the serotonin transporter number in the striatum.
   E. None of the above.

The correct response is option A.

Postmortem brain tissue studies of young (5- to 29-year-old) and older (62- to 84-year-old) subjects have shown that the major midbrain serotonin neuronal population of the median raphe does not show alterations in the amount of the synthetic enzyme tryptophan hydroxylase with increasing age.

Recent PET imaging studies of 5-HT_{1A} receptor binding in living subjects reported a 10% decrease in binding per decade for this serotonin receptor subtype, as well as a 17% per decade loss of 5-HT_{2A} receptors in a variety of brain regions from age 20 to middle age than at later ages. Others have reported decreased serotonin transporter number in the striatum (6.6% per decade) and 3%–4% per decade decrease in other serotonin transporter–rich regions with increasing age when SPECT imaging techniques were used. **(pp. 92–93)**

5.4   Brain corticotropin-releasing factor (CRF) concentrations are noted to be

   A. Increased in frontal and temporal cortex of postmortem brains of patients with Alzheimer's disease compared to controls.
   B. Increased in nucleus basalis and hypothalamus in patients with Alzheimer's disease.
   C. Either unchanged, increased, or decreased in cerebrospinal fluid (CSF) from subjects with Alzheimer's disease, depending on the study cited.
   D. Poor diagnostic markers of dementia severity in Alzheimer's disease.
   E. None of the above.

The correct response is option C.

CSF concentrations of CRF in clinical Alzheimer's disease have been reported to be either unchanged or decreased.

Concentrations of CRF were reported to be decreased in frontal and temporal cortex of postmortem Alzheimer's disease brain relative to age-matched non-Alzheimer's disease control tissues in 1985. CRF concentrations in the Alzheimer's disease group were not altered in subcortical regions such as the nucleus basalis or hypothalamus. The presence of significant CRF cortical deficits may become an important therapeutic target and diagnostic marker for Alzheimer's disease; CRF deficits may precede those that occur in other neurotransmitters. **(pp. 98–100)**

5.5   Which of the following statements is true?

   A. Somatostatin and acetylcholine changes in Alzheimer's disease occur sometime after CRF loss.
   B. Nitric oxide has been hypothesized to contribute to oxidative damage at the cellular level in Alzheimer's disease.
   C. Somatostatin levels may increase with age.
   D. A and B.
   E. A, B, and C.

The correct response is option D.

Somatostatin and acetylcholine changes in Alzheimer's disease apparently occur sometime after CRF loss, and they may interact. In Alzheimer's disease, nitric oxide has been hypothesized to contribute to oxidative damage that results at the cellular level during the neurodegenerative process. Somatostatin levels may decrease with age, and this decrease may be partially reversible with application of growth factors. **(pp. 101–102)**

C h a p t e r   6

Genetics

Select the single best response for each question.

6.1   The following are all examples of genes on which loci for Alzheimer's disease are found *except*

    A. Chromosome 1.
    B. Chromosome 14.
    C. Chromosome 19.
    D. Chromosome 21.
    E. Chromosome 24.

The correct response is option E.

Loci for Alzheimer's disease have not been found on chromosome 24.

    The first identified autosomal dominant gene was the beta-amyloid precursor protein *(APP)* gene located on chromosome 21 (Goate et al. 1991). A second Alzheimer's disease locus was found on chromosome 14 (Schellenberg et al. 1992; St. George-Hyslop et al. 1992) and is now called presenilin-1 *(PS1)*. A third Alzheimer's disease gene has been localized to chromosome 1 and termed presenilin-2 *(PS2)*. In 1991, Pericak-Vance and colleagues reported linkage of disease to a locus on chromosome 19 in families with late-onset Alzheimer's disease. **(pp. 110–111)**

6.2   Which of the following statements is true of purported loci, genes, and mutations associated with Alzheimer's disease?

    A. The pathogenic mechanisms of *APP*, *PS1*, and *PS2* mutations are completely understood.
    B. Mutations appear to be associated with decreased production of the long form of beta-amyloid.
    C. Mutations appear to be associated with increased production of the short form of beta-amyloid.
    D. The short form of beta-amyloid is less pathogenic than the long form.
    E. The long form of beta-amyloid is less pathogenic than the short form.

The correct response is option D.

The short form of beta-amyloid is less pathogenic than the long form.

    The pathogenic mechanisms of the *APP*, *PS1*, and *PS2* mutations are not completely understood, but each appears to be associated with increased production of the long form of beta-amyloid (beta-amyloid 42), relative to the production of the shorter forms (mostly beta-amyloid 40) of beta-amyloid (Hardy 1997). **(p. 113)**

6.3   Frontotemporal dementia (FTD) has been the focus of genetic investigations in recent years because approximately what percentage of those with FTD have a family history of the disorder?

    A. 20%.
    B. 30%.
    C. 40%.
    D. 50%.
    E. 70%.

The correct response is option D.

Frontotemporal dementia (FTD) has been the focus of genetic investigations in recent years because approximately 50% of those with FTD have a family history of the disorder (Neary 2000). **(p. 113)**

6.4   In Parkinson's disease, genetics point to which of the following?

    A. Some evidence indicates that, parallel to Alzheimer's disease, age at onset is inherited.
    B. Replication studies have consistently confirmed candidate genes under study.
    C. Genes identified to date have dissimilar mechanisms of action.
    D. Ubiquitin proteasome pathway is not thought to be figurative in cell death.
    E. The mode of inheritance appears to be similar among the loci.

The correct response is option A.

The genetics of Parkinson's disease parallel the genetics of Alzheimer's disease in several ways. Evidence indicates that the age at onset of Parkinson's disease is inherited (Li et al. 2002; Zareparsi et al. 2002).

    There appear to be multiple susceptibility genes that may increase the risk of developing Parkinson's disease; however, replication studies have not consistently confirmed any of the candidate genes under study. The genes identified to date appear to have a common mechanism, as all play a critical role in disrupting protein folding and degradation through the ubiquitin proteasome pathway, which then leads to cell death (Mouradian 2002). **(pp. 113–114)**

6.5   Genetics of depression in the elderly include all of the following *except*

    A. More men of a depressed group with short alleles of the serotonin transporter–linked polymorphic region *(5HTTLPR)* as compared to controls.
    B. Those elderly with short alleles showed a more rapid reduction in Hamilton Rating Scale for Depression when treated with paroxetine, as compared to those with long alleles.
    C. Depressed elderly individuals carrying at least one *APOE* epsilon 4 had white matter intensities on MRI scans.
    D. There is an association between subcortical gray matter hyperintensities and presence of at least one *APOE* epsilon 4 allele.
    E. There has not been a consistent relation between *APOE* epsilon 4 allele and late-life depression.

The correct response is option B.

The *5HTTLPR* gene may affect response to antidepressant medications among elderly control subjects. In a group of elderly patients taking paroxetine and nortriptyline, on average, those with the long allele genotype showed a more rapid reduction in Hamilton Rating Scale for Depression score than did those with a short allele, despite equivalent paroxetine concentrations (Pollock et al. 2000).

    In the study by Steffens et al. (2003), 23% of depressed men had two short alleles, compared with only 5% of the male control subjects. In a group weighted with elderly individuals carrying at least one *APOE* epsilon 4 allele, those with depressive symptoms reported on the Geriatric Depression Scale had more white matter intensities on MRI scans (Nebes et al. 2001). An association between subcortical gray matter hyperintensities and presence of at least one *APOE* epsilon 4 allele in elderly patients with major depression has been reported by Steffens et al. **(pp. 114–115)**

References

Goate A, Chartier-Harlin MC, Mullan M, et al: Segregation of a missense mutation in the amyloid precursor protein gene with familial Alzheimer's disease. Nature 349:704–706, 1991

Hardy J: Amyloid, the presenilins and Alzheimer's disease. Trends Neurosci 20:154–159, 1997

Li Y, Scott WK, Hedges DJ, et al: Age at onset in two common neurodegenerative diseases is genetically controlled. Am J Hum Genet 70:985–993, 2002

Mouradian MM: Recent advances in the genetics and pathogenesis of Parkinson disease. Neurology 58:179–185, 2002

Neary D: Frontotemporal dementia, in Dementia. Edited by O'Brien J, Ames D, Burns A. London, Arnold, 2000, pp 737–746

Nebes RD, Vora IJ, Meltzer CC, et al: Relationship of deep white matter hyperintensities and apolipoprotein E genotype to depressive symptoms in older adults without clinical depression. Am J Psychiatry 158:878–884, 2001

Pericak-Vance MA, Bebout JL, Gaskell PC, et al: Linkage studies in familial Alzheimer disease: evidence for chromosome 19 linkage. Am J Hum Genet 48:1034–1050, 1991

Pollock BG, Ferrell RE, Mulsant BH, et al: Allelic variation in the serotonin transporter promoter affects onset of paroxetine treatment response in late-life depression. Neuropsychopharmacology 23:587–590, 2000

Schellenberg GD, Bird TD, Wijsman EM, et al: Genetic linkage evidence for a familial Alzheimer's disease locus on chromosome 14. Science 258:668–671, 1992

St. George-Hyslop P, Haines J, Rogaev E, et al: Genetic evidence for a novel familial Alzheimer's disease locus on chromosome 14. Nat Genet 2:330–334, 1992

Steffens DC, Trost WT, Payne ME, et al: Apolipoprotein E genotype and subcortical vascular lesions in older depressed patients and control subjects. Biol Psychiatry 54:674–681, 2003

Zareparsi S, Camicioli R, Sexton G, et al: Age at onset of Parkinson disease and apolipoprotein E genotypes. Am J Med Genet 107:156–161, 2002

C h a p t e r   7

Psychological Aspects of Normal Aging

Select the single best response for each question.

7.1   Memory aging research has shown that

A. Age-related declines tend to increase as the environmental support provided by the task decreases.
B. Age-related declines are more evident in recall tasks than in recognition tasks.
C. Significant age-related decline occurs in the capacity of primary memory.
D. A and B.
E. A, B, and C.

The correct response is option D.

A general theme of memory aging research is that age-related declines tend to increase as the environmental support provided by the task decreases. Age-related declines in memory performance are more evident in recall tasks, which involve self-directed retrieval, than in recognition tasks.

The capacity of primary memory (e.g., digit span) is relatively constant as a function of age, whereas a significant age-related decline occurs in the capacity of secondary memory. **(pp. 122–123)**

7.2   Communication abilities of older adults show all of the following changes *except*

A. Substantial age-related deficits in discourse, text, or prose processing.
B. Level of education and verbal intelligence could account for some portion of the observed age effect on text recall performance.
C. Traditional laboratory-based problem-solving tasks do not seem to be predictive of everyday problem-solving performances for older adults.
D. Older adults have been shown to have deficits in auditory processing in laboratory settings.
E. Older adults do not seem to have disproportionate problems in processing everyday conversations or spoken input from television or radio.

The correct response is option C.

Traditional laboratory-based problem-solving tasks seem to be predictive of everyday problem-solving performances for older adults.

Earlier studies showed substantial age-related deficits in discourse, text, or prose processing among older adults. The level of education and verbal intelligence could account for some portion of the observed age effects on text recall performance. Older adults have been shown to have deficits in auditory processing in laboratory settings; however, older adults do not seem to have disproportionate problems in processing everyday conversations or spoken input from television or radio. **(pp. 122–124)**

7.3   Neuroimaging studies of normal older adults show

    A. Preferential deterioration of right-hemisphere structures.
    B. Generalized brain atrophy and decreases in resting cerebral blood flow with advanced age.
    C. Demyelination of subcortical, periventricular brain structures is rare in aging.
    D. No selective frontal lobe decline in the aging brain.
    E. Unchanged frontal lobe blood flow.

The correct response is option B.

Whereas generalized brain atrophy and decreases in resting cerebral blood flow with advanced age have been commonly noted (Raz 2000), some investigators report particularly pronounced reductions in frontal lobe blood flow (Gur et al. 1987) and volume (Coffey et al. 1992; Raz et al. 1997) in older adults.

Neuroanatomical and neuroimaging studies of normal older adults failed to show preferential deterioration of right-hemisphere structures. Demyelination of subcortical, periventricular brain structures is common in aging and is associated with signs of frontal lobe deficits on neuropsychological examination. Histopathological studies show selective frontal lobe decline in the aging brain. **(pp. 124–125)**

7.4   Research on intellectual functioning has shown which of the following?

    A. Fluid abilities tend to remain stable over the adult life span.
    B. Cognition and functional capacities are not closely related.
    C. Alzheimer's disease is projected to quadruple every 5 years after age 65.
    D. Studies from around the world have shown that about a quarter to a third of living centenarians may have dementia.
    E. Compared with other illnesses such as type II diabetes or diastolic hypertension, age itself is the strongest predictor of performing at or below the twenty-fifth percentile on a battery of neuropsychological tests.

The correct response is option E.

Age itself is the strongest factor for performing at or below the twenty-fifth percentile on a battery of neuropsychological tests.

Crystallized abilities, or knowledge acquired in the course of the socialization process, tend to remain stable over the adult life span, whereas fluid abilities, or abilities involved in the solution of novel problems, tend to decline gradually from younger to older adulthood. Cognition and functional capacities are closely related, with age, health, and diseases as potential contributing factors. Prevalence of dementia of the Alzheimer's type is projected to double every 5 years after age 65, and 360,000 new cases will occur each year. Centenarian studies from around the world (Poon 2001) have shown that about a quarter to a third of living centenarians may *not* have dementia and have maintained significant cognitive functions. **(pp. 126–127)**

7.5   Regarding the personality structure of the elderly,

    A. It has been shown to have remarkable stability over long periods of the life span.
    B. There are declines on dimensions of neuroticism.
    C. There are increases on dimensions of openness to experience.
    D. A and B.
    E. A and C.

The correct response is option D.

The American pattern of declines on the dimensions of neuroticism, extraversion, and openness to experience and increases in agreeableness and conscientiousness was consistently replicated in various cultures and nations, suggesting that these cross-sectional age differences were due to intrinsic maturational processes.

Contrary to popular conceptions that personality changes dramatically throughout adulthood, several longitudinal studies have shown remarkable stability over long periods of the life span. **(pp. 127–128)**

7.6   Which of the following is *not* true of coping in later life?

A. Older people have lower levels of internal control.
B. Religious affiliation and strong spiritual beliefs serve to offset and buffer negative effects of some life experiences.
C. Minority groups express greater satisfaction in using religion as a coping strategy.
D. Religious beliefs and practices could be related to lower levels of depression.
E. Older persons have less emotional reactivity when faced with stress than do younger adults.

The correct response is option A.

Researchers have found that older persons have higher levels of internal control and less emotional reactivity when faced with stress than do younger adults.

Findings show that religious affiliation and involvement and strong spiritual beliefs serve to offset and buffer the negative effects of some life experiences, such as health problems that are experienced in later life. Neighbors et al. (1983) reported that marginalized minority groups, unlike whites, used more religious coping when faced with problems, and they expressed greater satisfaction in using religion as a coping strategy. Although the evidence is mixed regarding the effects of religiosity and spirituality on physical and emotional health outcomes, some research suggests that religious beliefs and practices are related to higher levels of well-being. **(pp. 128–129)**

7.7   Research on caregiving has shown that

A. Depression and burden are higher among white caregivers than among African American caregivers.
B. Depression and burden are higher among white caregivers than among Hispanic caregivers.
C. Telephone interventions are not particularly effective for elderly persons.
D. African American caregivers tend to use less positive appraisal than white caregivers.
E. African American caregivers who appraised greater caregiving rewards were most likely to have higher levels of education.

The correct response is option A.

Findings show that depression and burden are higher among white caregivers than among African American caregivers, depression is similar between white caregivers and Hispanic caregivers, and burden is similar between Hispanic caregivers and African American caregivers.

Telephone interventions have been found to be increasingly effective and are well suited to elderly persons for whom transportation to sites of care is often a problem. Other evidence (Hinrichsen and Ramirez 1992) has shown that African American and white caregivers had similar use of appraisal when faced with stressful caregiving situations. Picot (1995) reported that African American caregivers who appraised greater caregiving rewards were most likely to be older and have lower levels of education. **(pp. 130–131)**

References

Coffey CE, Wilkinson WE, Parashos IA, et al: Quantitative cerebral anatomy of the aging human brain: a cross-sectional study using magnetic resonance imaging. Neurology 42:527–536, 1992

Gur RC, Gur RE, Obrist WD, et al: Age and regional cerebral blood flow at rest and during cognitive activity. Arch Gen Psychiatry 44:617–621, 1987

Hinrichsen GA, Ramirez M: Black and white dementia caregivers: a comparison of their adaptation, adjustment, and service utilization. Gerontologist 32:375–381, 1992

Neighbors HW, Jackson JS, Bowman PJ, et al: Stress, coping, and Black mental health: preliminary findings from a national study. Prev Hum Serv 2:5–29, 1983

Picot S: Choice and social exchange theory and the rewards of African American caregivers. J Natl Black Nurses Assoc 7:29–40, 1994

Poon LW: Centenarians, in The Encyclopedia of Aging, 3rd Edition. Edited by Maddox GL, Atchley RC, Evans JG, et al. New York, Springer, 2001, pp 179–180

Raz N: Aging of the brain and its impact on cognitive performance: integration of structural and functional findings, in The Handbook of Aging and Cognition, 2nd Edition. Edited by Craik FIM, Salthouse TA. Mahwah, NJ, Lawrence Erlbaum, 2000, pp 1–90

Raz N, Gunning FM, Head D, et al: Selective aging of the human cerebral cortex observed in vivo: differential vulnerability of the prefrontal gray matter. Cereb Cortex 7:268–282, 1997

Chapter 8

Social and Economic Factors Related to Psychiatric Disorders in Late Life

Select the single best response for each question.

8.1   Evidence concerning the relation between race and psychiatric morbidity of the elderly demonstrates that
    A. Race differences in depressive symptoms among the elderly are clear-cut.
    B. Older Hispanics appear to report higher levels of depressive symptoms than do whites or African Americans.
    C. There is a higher prevalence of alcohol and drug abuse among whites.
    D. There is a consistently higher level of depressive symptoms in African Americans than among whites.
    E. None of the above.

The correct response is option B.

Although evidence is scant, older Hispanics appear to report higher levels of depressive symptoms than do either whites or African Americans.

   Evidence concerning the relation between race/ethnicity and psychiatric morbidity is mixed. Race differences in depressive symptoms among the elderly are not clear-cut. Race differences are rarely observed in studies based on diagnostic measures, with the exception of a higher prevalence of alcohol and drug abuse among nonwhites. **(pp. 143–144)**

8.2   In general, all of the following are true *except*
    A. High levels of psychiatric symptoms are strongly related to low levels of education.
    B. Socioeconomic status and education in particular are weaker predictors of psychiatric symptoms in late life than at younger ages.
    C. Retirement increases the risk of psychiatric disorders.
    D. Women who have been widowed more than once are at greater risk for depression than those widowed only once.
    E. No evidence indicates that childbearing history is related to psychiatric status during later life.

The correct response is option C.

No evidence indicates that retirement increases the risk of psychiatric disorders.

   In general, high levels of psychiatric symptoms are strongly related to low levels of education. Some evidence suggests that socioeconomic status in general, and education in particular, is a weaker predictor of psychiatric symptoms in late life than at younger ages. Not surprisingly, perhaps, women who have been widowed more than once are at greater risk for depression than those widowed only once. No evidence indicates that childbearing history is related to psychiatric status during later life. Indeed, children are a major source of social support for most older adults. **(pp. 143–145)**

8.3   Church attendance and participation in other religious activities are associated with a decreased risk of

A. Alcohol abuse.
B. Depression.
C. Anxiety.
D. A and B.
E. A, B, and C.

The correct response is option E.

Social integration may protect individuals from psychiatric disorder. A growing body of research suggests that church attendance and participation in other religious activities are associated with a decreased risk of psychiatric morbidity, including alcohol abuse, depression, and anxiety disorders. **(p. 145)**

8.4   Risk factors for psychiatric disorders in late life include all of the following *except*

A. Chronic physical illnesses.
B. Cognitive impairment.
C. Perceived poor health.
D. Disability as measured in terms of activities of daily living impairment.
E. Lack of substantial social network size.

The correct response is option E.

Most studies have failed to show significant relations between social network size or structure and risk of depression.
     In addition to chronic physical illnesses, an increased risk of depression during late life is associated with other health indicators, including cognitive impairment (Blazer et al. 1991), perceived poor health (Henderson et al. 1993), and disability, measured in terms of activities of daily living impairment. **(pp. 145–146)**

8.5   Recovery from depression is

A. Affected by the presence of a confidant.
B. Affected by social network size.
C. Affected by perception of high-quality support.
D. Unrelated to religious participation.
E. More strongly predicted by the clinical features of the index episode than by social factors.

The correct response is option C.

Perception of high-quality support seems to significantly increase the likelihood of recovery.
     To date, no evidence shows that the presence of a confidant affects the likelihood of recovery from depression. Results are contradictory with regard to the relation between size of social network and probability of recovery from a depressive episode. One form of social integration, religious

participation, has been shown to predict recovery from major depression. Social factors were stronger predictors of outcome than were the clinical features of the index episode, although large proportions of variance remained unexplained. **(pp. 151–152)**

8.6   Among older alcoholics, more favorable outcomes were associated with

A. Female gender.
B. Higher socioeconomic status.
C. White race.
D. Being married, especially among men.
E. All of the above.

The correct response is option E.

Helzer and colleagues (1984) reported that among older alcoholic persons, more favorable outcomes were associated with female gender, white race, and higher socioeconomic status. Bailey et al. (1965) reported that being married increases the likelihood of recovery, especially among older men. **(p. 153)**

8.7   Mental health service use by the elderly has shown all of the following *except*

A. Women are more likely to seek care for psychiatric problems.
B. Gender is related to volume of care received.
C. Older patients, ages 65 and older, are less likely to seek mental health treatment than those ages 25–64.
D. Only age is a significant predictor of both receipt and volume of care.
E. Need factors are not significant predictors of volume of care received.

The correct response is option B.

Gender is unrelated to the volume of care received.

Women are more likely to seek care for psychiatric problems. Interestingly, only age is a significant predictor of both receipt and volume of care. Both older (ages 65 and older) and younger adults (ages 18–24) are less likely to seek mental health treatment than those ages 25–64, and when treatment is received, the older and younger adults obtain less care. **(pp. 153–154)**

8.8   Which of the following statements about older adults seeking outpatient care for mental health problems is true?

A. Most receive diagnoses and treatment in the general medical sector.
B. Older adults are far less likely than the middle aged to receive mental health treatment from psychiatrists.
C. Eighty percent of all older adults with primary or secondary psychiatric diagnoses receive treatment by primary care physicians.
D. A and B.
E. A, B, and C.

The correct response is option E.

Most older adults seeking outpatient care for mental health problems receive diagnoses and treatment in the general medical sector. Older adults are twice as likely to receive mental health treatments from general medical providers than from specialty mental health providers. Schurman et al. (1985) reported that 80% of all older adults with primary or secondary psychiatric diagnoses received treatment by primary care physicians. Data from the 1989 and 1990 National Ambulatory Medical Care Surveys indicated that both old and young adults were far less likely than the middle aged to receive mental health treatment from psychiatrists (Schappert 1993). **(p. 155)**

References

Bailey M, Haberman P, Alksne H: The epidemiology of alcoholism in an urban residential area. Q J Stud Alcohol 26:19–40, 1965

Blazer DG, Burchett B, Service C, et al: The association of age and depression among the elderly: an epidemiologic exploration. J Gerontol 46:M210–M215, 1991

Helzer JE, Carey KE, Miller RH: Predictors and correlates of recovery in older versus younger alcoholics, in Nature and Extent of Alcohol Problems Among the Elderly. Edited by Maddox G, Robins LN, Rosenberg N. Rockville, MD, National Institute on Alcohol Abuse and Alcoholism, 1984, pp 83–99

Henderson AS, Jorm AF, MacKinnon A, et al: The prevalence of depressive disorders and the distribution of depressive symptoms in later life: a survey using draft ICD-10 and DSM-III-R. Psychol Med 23:719–729, 1993

Schappert SM: Office visits to psychiatrists: United States, 1989–1990. Adv Data 237:1–16, 1993

Schurman RA, Kramer PD, Mitchell JB: The hidden mental health network. Arch Gen Psychiatry 42:89–94, 1985

Chapter 9

The Psychiatric Interview of Older Adults

Select the single best response for each question.

9.1   The psychiatric interview of older adults can be complicated by

    A. Their not equating present distress with past episodes that are symptomatically similar.

    B. Their becoming angry or irritated when a clinician continues to probe previous periods of overt disability in usual activities.

    C. Their having experienced a major illness or trauma in childhood but viewing this information as being of no relevance to the present episode.

    D. A histrionic personality style.

    E. All of the above.

The correct response is option E.

Unfortunately, the older adult may not equate present distress with past episodes that are symptomatically similar, so the perspective of the family is especially valuable in the attempt to link current and past episodes. An older person sometimes becomes angry or irritated when the clinician continues to probe. Not infrequently, the older adult has experienced a major illness or trauma in childhood or as a younger adult, but he or she views this information as being of no relevance to the present episode and therefore dismisses it. Older persons who have chronic and moderately severe anxiety or a histrionic personality style—as well as distressed patients with Alzheimer's disease— tolerate their symptoms poorly. **(p. 167)**

9.2   Medication history of the older adult

    A. Should involve having the older person bring in all pill bottles.

    B. Should involve a double check between the written schedule and pill containers.

    C. Should assess alcohol intake.

    D. Should assess substance abuse.

    E. All of the above.

The correct response is option E.

The clinician should ask the older person to bring in all pill bottles as well as a list of medications taken and the dosage schedule. A double check between the written schedule and the pill containers will frequently expose some discrepancy. Older persons are less likely than younger persons to abuse alcohol, but a careful history of alcohol intake is essential to the diagnostic workup. Substance abuse beyond alcohol and prescription drugs is rare in older adults, but not entirely absent. **(pp. 167–168)**

9.3   Evaluation of the family of the psychiatrically ill older adult would include all of the following parameters of support *except*

A. Availability of the family member.
B. Tangible services provided by the family.
C. Patient's perception of family support.
D. Tolerance by the family of specific behaviors derived from the psychiatric disorder.
E. Consideration of only those individuals genetically related to the patient.

The correct response is option E.

For clinical purposes, the family consists not only of individuals genetically related but also of those who have developed relationships and are living together as if they were related.

At least four parameters of support are important for the clinician to evaluate as the treatment plan evolves. These include 1) availability of family members to the older person over time, 2) the tangible services provided by the family to the disturbed older person, 3) the perception of family support by the older patient (and subsequently the willingness of the patient to cooperate and accept support), and 4) tolerance by the family of specific behaviors that derive from the psychiatric disorder. **(pp. 168–169)**

9.4   Examples of depressive delusions would be least likely to involve which of the following statements?

A. "I've lost my mind."
B. "My body is disintegrating."
C. "I ought to be executed."
D. "I have an incurable illness."
E. "I have caused some great harm."

The correct response is option C.

Of 161 patients with endogenous depression studied by Meyers and colleagues (Meyers and Greenberg 1986; Meyers et al. 1985), 72 (45%) were found to be delusional as determined by Research Diagnostic Criteria). These delusions included beliefs such as "I've lost my mind," "My body is disintegrating," "I have an incurable illness," and "I have caused some great harm." **(p. 170)**

9.5   Barriers to effective communication between the older patient and clinician can include

A. Physician perceiving the older adult patient incorrectly because of personal fears of aging and death.
B. The patient's perceptual problems.
C. Patient taking longer to respond to inquiries, resisting the physician who attempts to hurry through the interview.
D. Patient perceiving the physician unrealistically.
E. All of the above.

The correct response is option E.

The clinician may perceive the older adult patient incorrectly because of personal fears of aging and death or because of previous negative experiences with his or her own parents. Perceptual problems, such as hearing and visual impairments, may exacerbate disorientation and complicate the communication of problems to the clinician. Elderly persons frequently take longer to respond to inquiries and resist the clinician who attempts to rush through the history-taking interview. The elderly patient may perceive the physician unrealistically, on the basis of previous life experiences (that is, transference may occur). **(p. 175)**

References

Meyers BS, Greenberg R: Late-life delusional depression. J Affect Disord 11:133–137, 1986

Meyers BS, Greenberg R, Varda M: Delusional depression in the elderly, in Treatment of Affective Disorders in the Elderly. Edited by Shamoian CA. Washington, DC, American Psychiatric Press, 1985, pp 37–63

Chapter 10

Use of the Laboratory in the Diagnostic Workup of Older Adults

Select the single best response for each question.

10.1 Serum vitamin B_{12} and folate levels

    A. Are rarely important in the evaluation of the elderly patient.
    B. May point to etiologies of a range of neuropsychiatric disturbances.
    C. Would not be thought etiologic if recorded as normal.
    D. Are not related to hyperhomocysteinemia.
    E. Are not related to one-carbon metabolism in brain tissue.

The correct response is option B.

Vitamin B_{12} and folate deficiencies may result in neuropsychiatric disturbances, including depression, psychosis, and cognitive deficits. Measurement of serum vitamin B_{12} and folate levels is an integral part of the laboratory evaluation as the prevalence of B_{12} deficiency increases with age: the deficiency is present in up to 15% of the elderly population. B_{12} deficiency may have various clinical signs, including macrocytic anemia and neuropathy. Serum homocysteine levels may serve as a functional indicator of B_{12} and folate status because vitamin B_{12} is needed to convert homocysteine to methionine in one-carbon metabolism in brain tissue. **(pp. 181–182)**

10.2 Approximately what percentage of persons admitted from the community to a geropsychiatry unit may have a urinary tract infection that may result in a delirium?

    A. 10%.
    B. 20%.
    C. 35%.
    D. 45%.
    E. 55%.

The correct response is option B.

Identification of a urinary tract infection is critical in the elderly population, particularly in those with dementia. Approximately 20% of people admitted from the community to a geropsychiatry unit may have a urinary tract infection, and in many cases it may result in a delirium; however, the condition improves with appropriate antibiotic treatment. **(p. 182)**

10.3 Lithium is most likely to demonstrate which of the following ECG changes?

 A. AV block.
 B. Prolonged PR interval.
 C. Sick sinus syndrome.
 D. Bradycardia.
 E. QTc prolongation.

The correct response is option C.

Lithium appears to most affect the sinus node, and even at therapeutic levels it may result in sick sinus syndrome or sinoatrial block, either of which may occur early or later in treatment. At higher levels, there have been reports of sinus arrest and asystole.

   Individuals with preexisting bundle branch block who take tricyclic antidepressants are at increased risk for AV block. Even therapeutic levels are associated with prolonged PR intervals and QRS complexes; these results may be more pronounced in elderly individuals as the incidence and severity of adverse drug reactions increase with age. Antipsychotics also result in ECG changes; about 25% of individuals receiving antipsychotics exhibit ECG abnormalities Although many of these changes have historically been considered benign, there is increased concern that prolongation of the QTc interval may contribute to potentially fatal ventricular arrhythmias, particularly torsades de pointes. **(pp. 182–183)**

10.4 *APOE* testing has shown that

 A. A homozygous epsilon 4/epsilon 4 genotype is diagnostic for Alzheimer's disease.
 B. It is valuable in modifying the disease course and influencing current supportive treatments for Alzheimer's disease.
 C. It predicts response to cholinesterase inhibitors.
 D. It lacks hierarchy of the alleles for prediction or risk for development of Alzheimer's disease.
 E. None of the above.

The correct response is option E.

Multiple epidemiological studies have documented that the presence of the epsilon 4 allele is a risk factor for Alzheimer's disease (Roses 1997). Additionally, the presence of epsilon 4 alleles increases the specificity of the diagnosis of Alzheimer's disease. Despite these associations, the presence of an epsilon 4 allele, even a homozygous epsilon 4/epsilon 4 genotype, is not diagnostic for Alzheimer's disease. Other causes of dementia would have to be explored as clinically indicated. *APOE* testing is not currently recommended to predict dementia risk in asymptomatic individuals. Current treatments for cognitive dysfunction are limited to cholinesterase inhibitors, but response to these drugs is not dependent on *APOE* status. **(p. 186)**

10.5 Which of the following statements about genetic testing is *not* true? Genetic testing

 A. Results in transient heightened anxiety and depression.
 B. Can possibly result in hopelessness.
 C. Results in job loss or lack of insurability.
 D. Proves to be a valuable tool with untapped potential.
 E. Is recommended to predict dementia risk in asymptomatic individuals.

The correct response is option E.

Testing can result in transient heightened anxiety and depression; in the long term, a positive test may result in hopelessness. The inappropriate release of information could result in job loss or lack of insurability. Genetic testing is a tool with much untapped potential. **(pp. 186–187)**

10.6   Differences between AIDS-related and Alzheimer's dementia include all of the following *except*

    A. Mild protein elevation of CSF in Alzheimer's disease.
    B. Mononuclear CSF pleocytosis in AIDS-related dementia.
    C. Neuropathies in AIDS-related dementia.
    D. Aphasia and other cortical deficits uncommon in AIDS-related dementia.
    E. Cortical dementia in Alzheimer's disease.

The correct response is option A.

Alzheimer's disease is not typically associated with CSF abnormalities. Mild protein elevation of CSF is instead present in AIDS-related dementia. **(p. 181, Table 10–1)**

Reference

Roses AD: A model for susceptibility polymorphisms for complex diseases: apolipoprotein E and Alzheimer disease. Neurogenetics 1:3–11, 1997

Chapter 11

Neuropsychological Assessment of Dementia

Select the single best response for each question.

11.1   The most common cause for cognitive change after age 50 is

A. Alzheimer's disease.
B. Frontotemporal dementia.
C. Normal aging of the nervous system.
D. Vascular dementia.
E. None of the above.

The correct response is option C.

By far the most common cause for cognitive change after age 50 is normal aging of the nervous system. Compared to young adults, older individuals show selective losses in functions related to the speed and efficiency of information processing. Particularly vulnerable are memory retrieval abilities, attentional capacity, executive skills, and divergent thinking, such as working memory and multitasking. **(p. 191)**

11.2   The differences underlying memory loss of normal aging and that of Alzheimer's disease include

A. Consolidation or storage of new information in long-term memory stores.
B. Efficient accessing of recently stored information.
C. Difficulty with visuospatial tasks.
D. A and B.
E. A, B, and C.

The correct response is option D.

Different mechanisms underlie the memory loss of aging and that of Alzheimer's disease. In Alzheimer's disease, it is suggested that the problems reside in the consolidation or storage of new information in long-term memory stores. In normal aging, the principal problem appears to be the efficient accessing of recently stored information. Besides memory problems, older adults without dementing disorders also show some decrements compared to younger cohorts on tests of visuoperceptual, visuospatial, and constructional functions. **(pp. 191–192)**

11.3   The leading cause of dementia in elderly persons is

   A. Vascular disease.
   B. Alzheimer's disease.
   C. Lewy body disease.
   D. Frontotemporal disease.
   E. Corticobasal degeneration.

The correct response is option B.

Alzheimer's disease is the leading cause of dementia in elderly persons. Alone or in combination with other nervous system disorders, Alzheimer's disease accounts for nearly 50%–75% of all cases in Western countries.

   The second most common cause of dementia, accounting for 15%–30% of cases, is vascular dementia, which includes disorders arising from either large- or small-vessel strokes. Far less common are the frontal lobe disorders, which include the now well-recognized disorders of frontotemporal dementia, Pick's disease, and forms of progressive aphasia. Lewy body dementia and related movement disorders of the basal ganglia—including Parkinson's disease, progressive supranuclear palsy, corticobasal degeneration, Huntington's disease, and multisystem atrophy—together account for 10% of the cases. **(pp. 192–193)**

11.4   The earliest manifestation of Alzheimer's disease is

   A. Rapid forgetting of new information after very brief delays.
   B. Expressive language difficulty.
   C. Visuospatial difficulty.
   D. Apraxia.
   E. Circumlocution.

The correct response is option A.

On formal neuropsychological testing, the memory problem of Alzheimer's disease is manifest as a rapid forgetting of new information after very brief delays.

   As the disease progresses, other areas of cognition are involved, reflecting the specific spread of neuropathological involvement to the lateral temporal areas, parietal cortex, and frontal neocortical areas. Prototypical changes occur in expressive language, visuospatial function, higher executive controls, and semantic knowledge. Visuospatial problems become more prominent in later stages of the illness, resulting in dressing apraxia, difficulty in recognizing objects or people, and problems in performing familiar motor acts. Word search and circumlocution tendencies are common in conversational speech, whereas speech comprehension itself is better preserved, as are all other fundamental elements of communication. **(p. 193)**

11.5   Patients with vascular dementia could be expected to show all of the following *except*

   A. Memory deficits often patchy in nature.
   B. Impaired recollection of some recent event but surprisingly good memory of some other event occurring during the same time frame.
   C. Flattened learning curve over repeated trials.
   D. Low recall performance as well as rapid forgetting.
   E. Recognition improving dramatically with a recognition format.

The correct response is option D.

Recall performance can be quite low—similar to Alzheimer's disease—but is typically without the rapid forgetting shown in Alzheimer's disease.

Memory is involved, but deficits are often patchy in nature. Patients may show impaired recollection of some recent event but show a surprising memory of some other event occurring during the same time frame. On formal neuropsychological testing, the pattern shown in results of memory testing is one of inefficient acquisition of new information, leading to a flattened learning curve over repeating trials. Finally, recognition improves dramatically with a recognition format, suggesting a primary difficulty in retrieval rather than in storage or consolidation of new information. (p. 195)

11.6 The frontal variant of frontotemporal dementia would be expected to manifest

    A. Mutism.
    B. Preservation of insight.
    C. Recent memory impairment.
    D. Changes in social behavior and personality.
    E. Complaint of word loss and restriction in expressive vocabulary.

The correct response is option D.

The frontal variant is primarily characterized by the changes in social behavior and personality, reflecting the orbitofrontal (ventromedial) basis of the underlying pathology.

Reduction in spontaneous speech is common and probably related to the extent of frontal/anterior cingulate involvement; however, mutism is rare. Patients' insight into their condition is impaired, usually early in the course of the disorder. Patients with semantic dementia complain of word loss and restriction in expressive vocabulary. (pp. 195–196)

11.7 What percentage of patients with Parkinson's disease are reported to have dementia?

    A. 5%–10%.
    B. 10%–20%.
    C. 20%–40%.
    D. 50%–60%.
    E. 70%–80%.

The correct response is option C.

Typically, only 20%–40% of patients with Parkinson's disease are reported to have dementia, and there is some evidence that younger age at onset is a risk factor for Parkinson's disease dementia. (p. 197)

11.8 Geriatric depression shows all of the following deficits *except*

    A. Impairments on tests sensitive to frontal lobe function.
    B. Difficulties on sustained and selective attention.
    C. Set shifting.
    D. Perseverative errors and intrusional tendencies.
    E. All cognitive impairments remitting with treatment.

The correct response is option E.

With treatment, not all the cognitive impairments associated with geriatric depression remit. In older patients, these continuing impairments may be due to the co-occurrence of another disease process, such as Alzheimer's disease or vascular dementia.

On formal neuropsychological testing, geriatric depressed patients show impairments on tests sensitive to frontal lobe function. Difficulties can be readily seen on tests of selective and sustained attention, verbal fluency, inhibitory control, and set shifting. Perseverative errors and intrusional tendencies, although common in patients with both disorders, are particularly common in depressed patients. **(pp. 198–199)**

Chapter 12

Cognitive Disorders

Select the single best response for each question.

12.1 Computed tomography (CT) and magnetic resonance imaging (MRI) can detect which of the following as potentially treatable causes of dementia?

A. Tumors.
B. Subdural hematomas.
C. Periventricular hyperintensities on T2-weighted images.
D. A and B.
E. A, B, and C.

The correct response is option D.

CT and MRI can detect potentially treatable intracranial mass lesions such as tumors or subdural hematomas and can also suggest the presence of normal-pressure hydrocephalus (NPH).

The frequently observed periventricular hyperintensities on T2-weighted images obtained with high-resolution magnetic resonance scanners continue to be of unknown significance. These periventricular changes have not been clearly demonstrated to be attributable to "microvascular disease," and their usefulness in differential diagnosis remains unclear. **(p. 209)**

12.2 Cognitive deficits of Alzheimer's disease correlate

A. With density of neurofibrillary tangles.
B. With hyperphosphorylated tau.
C. With density of neuritic plaques.
D. A and B.
E. A and C.

The correct response is option D.

The major constituent of neurofibrillary tangles is a hyperphosphorylated form of the microtubule-associated phosphoprotein tau. The correlation between the density of postmortem neurofibrillary tangles and antemortem cognitive deficits is more robust than that between neuritic plaques and cognitive deficits. **(p. 213)**

12.3 Serotonin abnormalities of Alzheimer's disease include

A. Loss of serotonergic neurons in brain stem raphe nuclei.
B. Decreased concentration of serotonin in brain tissue.
C. Decreased concentration of serotonin in CSF.
D. Decreased serotonin receptor concentrations.
E. All of the above.

The correct response is option E.

In patients with Alzheimer's disease, there is a clear deficiency in brain serotonin systems, manifested by loss of serotonergic neurons in the brain stem raphe nuclei, decreased concentrations of serotonin and its metabolite in brain tissue and CSF, and decreased serotonin receptor concentrations. **(p. 214)**

12.4   Brain presynaptic cholinergic deficit has *not* been demonstrated in which of the following?

    A. Alzheimer's disease.
    B. Frontotemporal dementia.
    C. Vascular dementia.
    D. Lewy body dementia.
    E. C and D.

The correct response is option B.

Brain presynaptic cholinergic deficit has not been demonstrated in frontotemporal dementia.

    Whitehouse and colleagues (1982) demonstrated extensive neuronal loss in the cholinergic nucleus basalis of Meynert in patients with Alzheimer's disease. A brain presynaptic cholinergic deficit has also been demonstrated in vascular dementia (Erkinjuntti et al. 2002) and dementia with Lewy bodies (E.K. Perry et al. 1994). **(pp. 215–216)**

12.5   Cholinesterase inhibitors are best conceptualized as drugs

    A. That stabilize cognition, activities of daily living, and behavioral function.
    B. That improve cognitive function greatly.
    C. Only indicated for mild to moderate stages of Alzheimer's disease.
    D. Contraindicated in the treatment of Lewy body dementia.
    E. Predominately associated with the side effect of sedation.

The correct response is option A.

They are best conceptualized as drugs that stabilize cognition, activities of daily living, and behavioral function and that slow clinical deterioration in Alzheimer's disease. Stabilization of cognition and functioning for approximately 1 year has been demonstrated with both galantamine and donepezil.

    A consensus is emerging that cholinesterase inhibitor therapy should be started as soon as Alzheimer's disease, dementia with Lewy bodies, vascular dementia, or mixed dementia becomes apparent and that treatment should be continued at least into moderately advanced stages of disease, provided the drug is well tolerated. As is the case with all cholinesterase inhibitors, gastrointestinal symptoms—particularly nausea and vomiting (CNS cholinergic effects) and diarrhea—are the most frequent adverse effects. **(p. 215)**

12.6   Vitamin E and selegiline have *not* been shown to

    A. Have beneficial effects on cognitive function per se.
    B. Delay nursing home placement.
    C. Delay progression to severe dementia.
    D. Be more effective in combination than either agent alone.
    E. Delay loss of basic activities of daily living.

The correct response is option A.

Vitamin E and selegiline have no beneficial effects on cognitive function per se.

The combination of vitamin E and selegiline was no more effective than either agent alone. Both vitamin E and selegiline were more effective than placebo in delaying deterioration to functional end points that included nursing home placement, progression to severe dementia, and substantial loss of basic activities of daily living or death. **(p. 216)**

12.7 Dementia with a cerebrovascular contribution

A. Is as common as Alzheimer's disease.
B. Is most frequently seen as pure vascular dementia.
C. Lowers the threshold for and increases the magnitude of dementia caused by Alzheimer's disease.
D. Is associated with an especially high prevalence and severity of dementia with infarcts in the basal ganglia, thalamus, or deep white matter.
E. C and D.

The correct response is option E.

Infarcts lower the threshold for and increase the magnitude of dementia caused by Alzheimer's disease. Infarcts in the basal ganglia, thalamus, or deep white matter are associated with an especially high prevalence and severity of dementia.

Vascular dementia is not as common as Alzheimer's disease. Mixed dementia is more common than previously believed and may make up 10%–30% of late-life dementia. **(pp. 218–219)**

12.8 Most forms of frontotemporal dementia involve

A. Neuronal cell loss.
B. Gliosis.
C. Pick bodies.
D. Abnormal function of tau protein.
E. Amyloidopathy.

The correct response is option D.

It is increasingly clear that abnormal function of the cytoskeletal protein tau ("taupathy") is a central feature of most forms of frontotemporal dementia. Frontotemporal atrophy and microscopic changes are present in Pick's disease; the latter include neuronal cell loss, gliosis, and the presence of massed cytoskeletal elements called Pick bodies. Additional tau mutations were soon described by others (Hutton et al. 1998). Because these tau mutations demonstrated that tau dysfunction is sufficient to cause neurodegenerative dementia even in the absence of brain amyloidopathy, there is increased interest in the role of tau abnormalities in the pathogenesis of the much more common dementia disorder of Alzheimer's disease. **(pp. 220–221)**

12.9 Hypothyroidism

A. Can produce a dementia accompanied by irritability, paranoid ideation, and depression.
B. Can produce a dementia for which aggressive thyroid replacement results in the patient's return to previous level of functioning.
C. Is similar to vitamin B_{12} deficiency dementia in that B_{12} replacement leads to remission of dementia.
D. A and B.
E. A, B, and C.

The correct response is option A.

Hypothyroidism classically produces a cognitive syndrome of dementia accompanied by irritability, paranoid ideation, and depression. Once the dementia is established, even aggressive thyroid replacement therapy does not result in a return to the patient's previous level of functioning. Anecdotal reports suggest that B_{12} replacement in dementia that is apparently secondary to B_{12} deficiency may produce some cognitive improvement, but dementia persists. **(p. 221)**

12.10 Delirium in the elderly

    A. Usually persists for months in those hospitalized for medical or surgical reasons.
    B. Rarely results in full resolution of symptoms in a short time.
    C. Is often the initial presentation of an underlying dementia.
    D. Could have an insidious onset.
    E. All of the above.

The correct response is option E.

Levkoff et al. (1992) demonstrated that incident delirium in elderly persons hospitalized for medical or surgical reasons usually persists for months. Full resolution of symptoms of delirium in a short time was the exception rather than the rule in this study. An episode of delirium often is the initial presentation of an underlying dementia. In the elderly, a delirium secondary to drugs or to illnesses such as renal failure may have an insidious onset. **(p. 222)**

References

Erkinjuntti T, Kurz A, Gauthier S, et al: Efficacy of galantamine in probable vascular dementia and Alzheimer's disease combined with cerebrovascular disease: a randomised trial. Lancet 359:1283–1290, 2002

Hutton M, Lendon CL, Rizzu P, et al: Association of missense and 5'-splice-site mutations in tau with the inherited dementia FTDP-17. Nature 393:702–705, 1998

Levkoff SE, Evans DA, Liptzin B, et al: Delirium: the occurrence and persistence of symptoms among elderly hospitalized patients. Arch Intern Med 152:334–340, 1992

Perry EK, Haroutunian V, Davis KL, et al: Neocortical cholinergic activities differentiate Lewy body dementia from classical Alzheimer's disease. Neuroreport 5:747–749, 1994

Whitehouse PJ, Price DL, Struble RG, et al: Alzheimer's disease and senile dementia: loss of neurons in the basal forebrain. Science 215:1237–1239, 1982

Chapter 13

Movement Disorders

Select the single best response for each question.

13.1 All of the following are features of Parkinson's disease *except*

A. Postural instability.
B. Prevalence increasing with age.
C. Lewy bodies in the cytoplasm of degenerating neurons.
D. Resting tremor attenuating at least transiently during voluntary movement, much like that of essential tremor.
E. Presentation with an akinetic form in which resting tremor is minimal.

The correct response is option D.

The resting tremor of Parkinson's disease typically attenuates at least transiently during voluntary movement of the affected extremity, such as when the patient picks up an object, and is to be distinguished from the postural, antigravity tremor observed in essential tremor.

Parkinson's disease is a chronic, progressive, neurodegenerative illness that produces rigidity, slowness of movement (bradykinesia), postural instability, and, often, tremor at rest. The prevalence of Parkinson's disease increases with age, with estimates of 1% at age 60 and up to 2.6% at age 85 or older (Mutch et al. 1986; Sutcliffe et al. 1985). Parkinson's disease is characterized pathologically by abnormal collections of proteins, called Lewy bodies, in the cytoplasm of degenerating neurons. **(p. 232)**

13.2 Synkinetic movement refers to

A. Resting tremor.
B. Cogwheel rigidity.
C. Involuntary resistance to passive movement of the extremities.
D. Voluntary movement of contralateral extremity bringing out rigidity in ipsilateral limb.
E. None of the above.

The correct response is option D.

Active, voluntary movement of the contralateral extremity (synkinetic movement) can bring out subtle rigidity in an ipsilateral limb. In patients with resting tremor, the combination of rigidity and tremor results in cogwheel rigidity—that is, a jerky resistance to passive movement. The stiffness or rigidity of Parkinson's disease is detected clinically by testing for involuntary resistance to passive movement of the extremities. Parkinson's disease can be divided into two clinical forms: 1) tremor-dominant Parkinson's disease, in which tremor at rest is a prominent feature, and 2) postural instability and gait disorder, or akinetic Parkinson's disease, in which resting tremor is minimal, if present at all, and patients exhibit earlier balance difficulty. **(p. 232)**

13.3   Side effects of dopamine agonists include which of the following?

    A. Hallucinations.
    B. Dyskinesias.
    C. Dystonia.
    D. A and B.
    E. A, B, and C.

The correct response is option E.

The side effects of dopamine agonists are similar to those of levodopa: hallucinations, dyskinesias (head bobbing and involuntary writhing or twisting movements of the extremities), and dystonia (muscle spasms) are the most common. **(p. 233)**

13.4   All of the following are features of progressive supranuclear palsy (PSP) *except*

    A. Vertical gaze palsy.
    B. Early postural instability.
    C. Axial rigidity greater than appendicular rigidity.
    D. Good response to levodopa.
    E. Sloppy eating.

The correct response is option D.

Unlike in Parkinson's disease, there is little or no response to levodopa therapy because of degeneration of secondary neurons downstream from the dopaminergic substantia nigra pars compacta neurons.

    Progressive supranuclear palsy (PSP), or Steele-Richardson-Olszewski syndrome, features Parkinsonism without prominent tremor, vertical gaze palsy, axial (midline) more than appendicular (arm and leg) rigidity, early postural instability, and poor response to levodopa. PSP is often associated with frequent falling, lack of eye contact, monotonous speech, sloppy eating, and slowed mentation. **(pp. 234–235)**

13.5   Which of the following is *not* true of essential tremor?

    A. It is the most prevalent movement disorder among the elderly.
    B. Prevalence increases with age.
    C. Frequency may decrease with age.
    D. Early on, tremor is absent at rest.
    E. Usually it is not associated with a family history of tremor.

The correct response is option E.

There is usually a clear family history of tremor, and often the tremor attenuates with alcohol use, a phenomenon that can contribute to development of alcoholism in susceptible individuals.

    Essential tremor is the most prevalent movement disorder among adults and elderly persons, affecting up to 2% of the general population. The prevalence of essential tremor increases with age, and in individuals older than 70 years, estimates of the prevalence of essential tremor range to more than 10%. A key feature of essential tremor, at least early on, is that the tremor is absent at rest, only occurring during action or when a posture is being held. **(p. 236)**

13.6   Which of the following attenuates essential tremor?

   A. Propranolol.
   B. Primidone.
   C. Alcohol.
   D. Deep brain stimulation of the ventral intermediate nucleus of the contralateral thalamus.
   E. All of the above.

The correct response is option E.

The mainstays of medical treatment for essential tremor are propranolol therapy and primidone therapy. Often the tremor attenuates with alcohol use. Deep brain stimulation targeting the ventral intermediate nucleus of the contralateral thalamus is sometimes helpful in medically refractory cases. **(p. 236)**

References

Mutch WJ, Dingwall-Fordyce I, Downie AW, et al: Parkinson's disease in a Scottish city. Br Med J (Clin Res Ed) 292:534–536, 1986

Sutcliffe RL, Prior R, Mawby B, et al: Parkinson's disease in the district of the Northampton Health Authority, United Kingdom: a study of prevalence and disability. Acta Neurol Scand 72:363–379, 1985

Chapter 1 4

Mood Disorders

Select the single best response for each question.

14.1   In contrast to low rates of major depression among older adults in the community, it has been estimated that up to what percentage of hospitalized elders fulfill criteria for a major depressive episode?

A. 6%.
B. 11%.
C. 16%.
D. 21%.
E. 31%.

The correct response is option D.

In contrast to low rates (1%) of major depression among older adults in the community, it has been estimated that, depending on the diagnostic scheme, up to 21% of hospitalized elders fulfill criteria for a major depressive episode, and an additional 20%–25% have a minor depression (Koenig et al. 1997). **(p. 242)**

14.2   Mortality among elderly patients is

A. Increased in older men with physical health problems and depression.
B. Increased among nursing home patients with depression.
C. Increased in previously hospitalized depressed women.
D. A and B.
E. A, B, and C.

The correct response is option E.

Older men with physical health problems and depression are significantly more likely to die than similarly aged, physically ill, nondepressed men. Among depressed women, mortality is twice the expected rate; among the men, it is three times the expected rate. Rovner and colleagues (1991) found greater death rates among elderly nursing home patients with depression. Several recent studies involving medically ill patients likewise found greater mortality among those with depression. **(p. 243)**

14.3   Studies of prognosis of late-life depression show all of the following *except*

A. Older adults differ from their middle-age counterparts in terms of recovery and remission.
B. Elders who have recovered appear to experience residual depressive symptoms.
C. Seventy percent of elderly patients with major depression treated with adequate antidepressant regimens recover from the index episode.
D. Older patients who have experienced one or more moderate to severe episodes of major depression may need to continue antidepressant therapy permanently to minimize relapse.
E. Physical illness and cognitive impairment are associated with a worse outcome.

The correct response is option A.

In terms of recovery and remission, older adults do not differ from their middle-aged counterparts.

If they do recover, however, elders appear to experience residual depressive symptoms. Most clinicians and clinical investigators report that more than 70% of elderly patients with major depression who are treated with antidepressant medication (at an adequate dose for a sufficient time) recover from the index episode of depression. Once an older patient has experienced one or more moderate to severe episodes of major depression, he or she may need to continue antidepressant therapy permanently, to minimize the risk of relapse. Physical illness, disability, cognitive impairment, and more severe depression are associated with worse outcomes. **(pp. 244–245)**

14.4 Bipolar disorder in the elderly may have all of the following characteristics *except*

A. Tendency toward more rapid recurrences late in the illness.
B. Stressful events more likely to precede early-onset mania than late-onset mania.
C. Increased cerebral vulnerability playing a stronger role than life events in precipitating late-onset mania.
D. Association with low rates of familial affective disorder.
E. Genetic factors weighing heavily in the etiology.

The correct response is option E.

Evidence that genetic factors weigh heavily in the etiology of bipolar disorders in late life is virtually nonexistent, although the biological nature of this disorder would suggest some genetic contribution.

In a review of records of a small number of untreated patients with severe and prolonged bipolar disorder, Cutler and Post (1982) found a tendency toward more rapid recurrences late in the illness, with decreasing periods of normality. Ameblas (1987) emphasized a relationship between life events and onset of mania, noting that stressful events were more likely to precede early-onset mania than late-onset mania. Likewise, Shulman (1989) stressed that increased cerebral vulnerability due to organic insults (stroke, head trauma, other brain insults) played a stronger role than life events in precipitating late-onset mania (a factor that may also play a role in treatment resistance). Young and Klerman (1992) emphasized the low rates of familial affective disorder. **(pp. 245–246)**

14.5 Late-onset psychotic depression is characterized by which of the following?

A. Individuals with delusional depression tend to be older and respond to ECT.
B. Delusions of guilt are more common than delusions of persecution or of having an incurable illness.
C. It is not associated with poor social support.
D. Focus on the abdomen is uncommon.
E. None of the above.

The correct response is option A.

Individuals with delusional depression tend to be older and to respond to ECT, as opposed to tricyclic antidepressants (TCAs).

Delusions of persecution or of having an incurable illness are more common than delusions associated with guilt. Psychotic depression also tends to be associated with poor social support and, not surprisingly, bipolar illness. Focus on the abdomen is common in an elderly patient with delusional or psychotic depression. **(pp. 248–249)**

14.6   Uncomplicated bereavement is usually considered to include virtually all symptoms of depression, with the exception of _____, and to last up to _____ months.

   A. Extreme feelings of worthlessness, 2 months.
   B. Extreme feelings of worthlessness, 6 months.
   C. Irritability and hostility, 2 months.
   D. Irritability and hostility, 6 months.
   E. Sensations of somatic distress, 6 months.

   The correct response is option A.

   Uncomplicated bereavement is usually characterized by a symptom picture of major depression, yet the syndrome is recognized by the older adult as normal for the occasion and does not seriously interfere with necessary functioning. In DSM-IV-TR, the category of uncomplicated bereavement is designated for virtually all symptoms of depression experienced during the first 2 months after the loss, with the possible exception of extreme feelings of worthlessness or active suicidal ideation; any person exhibiting the full symptom picture of major depression at least 2 months after the death is considered to have a major depressive disorder warranting treatment. **(p. 250)**

14.7   Reversible dementia due to depression

   A. Predicts poor response to treatment of the depression.
   B. Is associated with patients attempting to conceal disabilities rather than highlighting them on formal mental status exam.
   C. Cannot be differentiated from that of bona fide dementia by way of REM sleep measures.
   D. Often indicates the presence of an early dementing illness.
   E. Should not be treated with a potent anticholinergic antidepressant such as imipramine.

   The correct response is option D.

   The combination of depression and reversible dementia in elderly patients often indicates the presence of an early dementing illness. In a study conducted by Reifler et al. (1982), elderly patients with depression and dementia, when treated with an antidepressant, responded with a remission of the depressive symptoms, while cognitive dysfunction persisted. The tendency among depressed patients is to highlight disabilities as opposed to concealing (or attempting to conceal) them. Dykierek and colleagues (1998) found that nearly all REM sleep measures differentiated significantly in patients with Alzheimer's disease, depressed elderly patients, and healthy controls. REM density, rather than REM sleep latency, was particularly important in separating depressed elders with dementia. Both depressed and nondepressed Alzheimer's patients were treated with the relatively potent anticholinergic antidepressant imipramine; patients improved whether or not they were in the treatment group, and cognitive function did not decline. **(p. 254)**

14.8   According to a recent study, what percentage of elders fulfill criteria for definite or questionable alcohol abuse?

   A. Between 2% and 4%.
   B. Between 3% and 6%.
   C. Between 10% and 15%.
   D. Between 20% and 30%.
   E. Between 30% and 40%.

   The correct response is option C.

Results of a recent study involving more than 10,000 older persons indicate that between 10% and 15% of elders fulfill criteria for definite or questionable alcohol abuse (Thomas and Rockwood 2001). **(p. 256)**

14.9   ECT

    A. Is less effective in older adults than in younger ones.

    B. Is no more effective than and has more side effects than antidepressants when used in the old-old populace.

    C. Has a relapse rate that may exceed 50% in the year after a course of ECT, without prophylaxis.

    D. Leads to a significant worsening of cognition in the majority of elderly depressed patients with dementia.

    E. Should be avoided in patients with cardiovascular, neurological, endocrine, or metabolic conditions.

The correct response is option C.

The relapse rate with no prophylactic intervention may exceed 50% in the year after a course of ECT. This relapse rate can be decreased if antidepressants or lithium carbonate is prescribed after the treatment. Investigators concluded that despite a higher level of physical illness and cognitive impairment, patients age 75 or older who had severe major depression tolerated ECT in a manner similar to the way in which younger patients tolerated the treatment, and the old-old patients demonstrated a similar or even better response. There is also evidence that ECT may be more effective and have fewer side effects than antidepressants when used to treat depression in old-old patients (Manly et al. 2000). Price and McAllister (1989) examined the efficacy of ECT in elderly depressed patients with dementia and found that only 21% experienced cognition problems; in most cases the problems were transient. Data do support the use of ECT in patients with cardiovascular, neurological, endocrine, or metabolic conditions, as well as a variety of other conditions (Stoudemire et al. 1998). **(pp. 261–262)**

References

Ameblas A: Life events and mania. Br J Psychiatry 150:235–240, 1987

Cutler NR, Post RM: Life course of illness in untreated manic-depressive patients. Compr Psychiatry 23:101–115, 1982

Dykierek P, Stadtmuller G, Schramm P, et al: The value of REM sleep parameters in differentiating Alzheimer's disease from old-age depression and normal aging. J Psychiatr Res 32:1–9, 1998

Koenig HG, George LK, Peterson BL, et al: Depression in medically ill hospitalized older adults: prevalence, characteristics, and course of symptoms based on six diagnostic schemes. Am J Psychiatry 154:1376–1383, 1997

Manly DT, Oakley SP Jr, Bloch RM: Electroconvulsive therapy in old-old patients. Am J Geriatr Psychiatry 8:232–236, 2000

Price TR, McAllister TW: Safety and efficacy of ECT in depressed patients with dementia: a review of clinical experience. Convuls Ther 5:61–74, 1989

Reifler BV, Larson E, Henley R: Coexistence of cognitive impairment and depression in geriatric outpatients. Am J Psychiatry 39:623–626, 1982

Rovner BW, German PS, Brant LJ, et al: Depression and mortality in nursing homes. JAMA 265:993–996, 1991

Shulman KI: The influence of age and aging on manic disorder. Int J Geriatr Psychiatry 4:63–65, 1989

Stoudemire A, Hill CD, Marquardt M, et al: Recovery and relapse in geriatric depression after treatment with antidepressants and ECT in a medical-psychiatric population. Gen Hosp Psychiatry 20:170–174, 1998

Thomas VS, Rockwood KJ: Alcohol abuse, cognitive impairment, and mortality among older people. J Am Geriatr Soc 49:415–420, 2001

Young RC, Klerman GL: Mania in late life: focus on age at onset. Am J Psychiatry 149:867–876, 1992

Chapter 15

Schizophrenia and Paranoid Disorders

Select the single best response for each question.

15.1 Factors distinguishing patients with very late onset schizophrenia from "true" schizophrenia of younger patients include all of the following *except*

A. Lower genetic load.
B. Less evidence of early childhood maladjustment.
C. Relative lack of formal thought disorder and negative symptoms.
D. Lesser risk of tardive dyskinesia.
E. Evidence of a neurodegenerative rather than a neurodevelopmental process.

The correct response is option D.

Factors distinguishing patients with very late onset schizophrenia from "true" schizophrenia patients include a lower genetic load, less evidence of early childhood maladjustment, a relative lack of thought disorder and negative symptoms (including blunted affect), greater risk of tardive dyskinesia, and evidence of a neurodegenerative rather than a neurodevelopmental process (Andreasen 1999; Howard et al. 1997). **(p. 271)**

15.2 What approximate percentage of Alzheimer's disease patients manifest psychotic symptoms, typically in the middle stages of the disease?

A. 10%–20%.
B. 15%–25%.
C. 25%–30%.
D. 35%–50%.
E. 55%–65%.

The correct response is option D.

Approximately 35%–50% of Alzheimer's disease patients manifest psychotic symptoms, typically in the middle stages of the disease. **(pp. 272–273)**

15.3   Alzheimer's disease patients with and without psychosis differ in all of the following *except*

A. Alzheimer's disease patients with psychosis show greater impairment in executive functioning.
B. Alzheimer's disease patients with psychosis have a greater prevalence of extrapyramidal signs.
C. Alzheimer's disease patients with psychosis have shown increased norepinephrine levels and reduced serotonin levels in subcortical regions.
D. Alzheimer's disease patients with psychosis typically warrant very long term maintenance therapy with antipsychotics.
E. Alzheimer's disease patients with psychosis have more prevalent behavioral disturbances such as agitation than hallucinations and paranoid delusions.

The correct response is option D.

Because psychotic symptoms in patients with dementia tend to remit in the late stages of the disease, very long term maintenance therapy with antipsychotics is typically unnecessary.

Alzheimer's disease patients with psychosis and those without psychosis differ in several important ways. Neuropsychologically, Alzheimer's disease patients with psychosis show greater impairment in executive functioning and a more rapid cognitive decline. Psychosis is associated with a greater prevalence of extrapyramidal signs in Alzheimer's disease. Neuropathologically, dementia patients with psychosis have shown increased neurodegenerative changes in the cortex, increased norepinephrine levels in subcortical regions, and reduced serotonin levels in both cortical and subcortical areas. Devanand and colleagues (1997) found that hallucinations and paranoid delusions were more persistent than depressive symptoms but less prevalent and less persistent than behavioral disturbances, particularly agitation. **(p. 273)**

15.4   Patients with dementia with Lewy bodies could be safely treated with all of the following *except*

A. Donepezil.
B. Quetiapine.
C. Rivastigmine.
D. Olanzapine.
E. Clozapine.

The correct response is option D.

Trials of olanzapine for Parkinson's disease–related dementia have indicated improvement of psychotic symptoms (Graham et al. 1998; Wolters et al. 1996) but exacerbation of parkinsonian symptoms (Goetz et al. 2000; Wolters et al. 1996).

Donepezil has also shown utility in treating paranoid and delusional ideation in patients who have dementia with Lewy bodies. Quetiapine appears to improve psychotic symptoms without worsening motor function. Clozapine has been shown to reduce symptoms and may improve tremor in some patients. **(p. 275)**

15.5   The most important risk factor for tardive dyskinesia is

A. Alcohol abuse.
B. Early extrapyramidal symptoms.
C. Certain ethnicities.
D. Aging.
E. None of the above.

The correct response is option D.

Aging appears to be the most important risk factor for tardive dyskinesia.

Previous investigators found tardive dyskinesia to be associated with early extrapyramidal symptoms, alcohol abuse or dependence, and certain ethnicities. **(pp. 275–276)**

References

Andreasen NC: I don't believe in late onset schizophrenia, in Late-Onset Schizophrenia. Edited by Howard R, Rabins PV, Castle DJ. Philadelphia, PA, Wrightson Biomedical, 1999, pp 111–123

Devanand DP, Jacobs DM, Tang MX, et al: The course of psychopathologic features in mild to moderate Alzheimer disease. Arch Gen Psychiatry 54:257–263, 1997

Goetz CG, Blasucci LM, Leurgans S, et al: Olanzapine and clozapine: comparative effects on motor function in hallucinating PD patients. Neurology 55:789–794, 2000

Graham JM, Sussman JD, Ford DS, et al: Olanzapine in the treatment of hallucinosis in idiopathic Parkinson's disease: a cautionary note. J Neurol Neurosurg Psychiatry 65:774–777, 1998

Howard R, Graham C, Sham P, et al: A controlled family study of late-onset non-affective psychosis (late paraphrenia). Br J Psychiatry 170:511–514, 1997

Wolters EC, Jansen ENH, Tuynman-Qua HG, et al: Olanzapine in the treatment of dopaminomimetic psychosis in patients with Parkinson's disease. Neurology 47:1085–1087, 1996

Chapter 16

Anxiety and Panic Disorders

Select the single best response for each question.

16.1 According to the Epidemiologic Catchment Area (ECA) study of the 1980s, the combined prevalence of phobia, panic disorder, and obsessive-compulsive disorder in people over age 65 is approximately what percentage?

A. 2.5%.
B. 3.5%.
C. 5.5%.
D. 6.5%.
E. 7%.

The correct response is option C.

The combined prevalence of phobia, panic disorder, and obsessive-compulsive disorder in people older than age 65 years was 5.5% according to the ECA study of the 1980s (Regier et al. 1990). **(p. 283)**

16.2 Panic disorder in those older than 65

A. Has a point prevalence of 0.4%.
B. Is not uncommonly ascribed to other causes by the elderly.
C. May present with fewer symptoms.
D. Is a relatively uncommon development in late life.
E. All of the above.

The correct response is option E.

In the ECA study, the point prevalence among middle-age subjects was 1.1%, whereas among those age 65 or older, the point prevalence was 0.4%. It is not uncommon for elderly adults to ascribe the symptoms to other causes, and the frequent waxing and waning of symptoms may make correct diagnosis difficult. Elderly individuals with late-onset panic attacks may have fewer symptoms and may do less to avoid the attacks. Development of panic disorder in late life is relatively uncommon, but it does occur. **(p. 284)**

16.3 In at least one study, what percentage of elderly Holocaust survivors met criteria for posttraumatic stress disorder more than 40 years after the war?

A. 10%.
B. 20%.
C. 30%.
D. 40%.
E. 50%.

The correct response is option E.

Nearly half of the elderly Holocaust survivors studied met criteria for posttraumatic stress disorder more than 40 years after the war (Kuch and Cox 1992). **(p. 286)**

16.4   The most common anxiety disorder of the elderly population is

A. Generalized anxiety disorder.
B. Posttraumatic stress disorder.
C. Social phobia.
D. Specific phobia.
E. Obsessive-compulsive disorder.

The correct response is option D.

Generalized anxiety disorder is the second most common anxiety disorder in the elderly population (phobias are the most common). **(p. 286)**

16.5   Which of the following factors could pertain to medical illnesses and anxiety among the elderly?

A. The older adult may worry about the effect and meaning of physical illness.
B. Anxiety may contribute to medical problems and complications.
C. Many anxiety symptoms may masquerade as medical illness.
D. Anxiety symptoms may be caused by medications given to elderly persons.
E. All of the above.

The correct response is option E.

There is a complex interaction among anxiety, medical illness, and the medications used to treat these conditions (Flint 1999). First, the older adult may have the realistic worry about the effect and meaning of physical illness. Anxiety may contribute to medical problems and complications. Medical illness may masquerade as anxiety symptoms. Many anxiety symptoms may masquerade as medical illness. Anxiety symptoms may be caused by the medications given to elderly persons to treat either physical or mental diseases. **(p. 287)**

16.6   Which of the following pharmacological agents has become the mainstay treatment of anxiety disorder in the elderly?

A. Tricyclic antidepressants (TCAs).
B. Monoamine oxidase inhibitors (MAOIs).
C. Selective serotonin reuptake inhibitors (SSRIs).
D. Benzodiazepines.
E. Buspirone.

The correct response is option C.

SSRIs have become the mainstay of anxiety disorder treatment, for several reasons. Fluoxetine has been shown to be effective in the treatment of depressed geriatric patients with agitation. Fluvoxamine and fluoxetine have been found to be effective for obsessive-compulsive disorder in clinical trials that have included some elderly patients. Case studies have shown sertraline, paroxetine, venlafaxine, fluoxetine, citalopram, and fluvoxamine to be effective in social phobias and anxiety. SSRIs have also been successfully used to treat posttraumatic stress disorder and specific phobias. Anxiety disorders and depressive disorders are frequently comorbid, and use of a single agent to treat both conditions decreases the rate of polypharmacy, a situation often occurring with the elderly. The side-effect profiles of SSRIs are much more acceptable than those of many older medications. (pp. 288–291)

References

Flint AJ: Anxiety disorders in late life. Can Fam Physician 45:2672–2679, 1999

Kuch K, Cox BJ: Symptoms of PTSD in 124 survivors of the Holocaust. Am J Psychiatry 149:337–340, 1992

Regier DA, Narrow WE, Rae DS: The epidemiology of anxiety disorders: the Epidemiologic Catchment Area (ECA) experience. J Psychiatr Res 24 (suppl 2):3–14, 1990

Chapter 17

Somatoform Disorders

Select the single best response for each question.

17.1   Somatization disorder is a psychiatric illness characterized by numerous physical complaints that are in excess of examination findings. This may be an especially challenging problem in the older patient with other chronic medical conditions. Which of the following is also true regarding somatization disorder?

   A. Paralleling the relative risk for depressive disorders, the risk for somatization disorder in women is twice that in men.
   B. Somatization disorder is common in patients with irritable bowel disease.
   C. As somatization disorder patients age, their reported symptoms tend to change and symptoms are reported in a less consistent pattern.
   D. Prominent pain symptoms are the typical "pseudoneurological" presentation.
   E. Another term for somatization disorder is Munchausen syndrome.

The correct response is option B.

Somatization disorder has been diagnosed in 42% of a sample of 50 medical outpatients with irritable bowel disease (Miller et al. 2001).

   Somatization disorder is seen almost exclusively in women and may have a prevalence rate ranging from 1% to 3%. The majority of individuals with somatization disorder demonstrate consistent symptom patterns as they age. Somatization disorder is characterized by multiple physical complaints that include pain at four or more sites, two gastrointestinal symptoms, one sexual symptom, and one pseudoneurological symptom (other than pain). Another term used to describe somatization disorder is Briquet's syndrome. **(p. 296)**

17.2   Undifferentiated somatoform disorder and hypochondriasis may present in the geriatric psychiatric patient. Distinguishing between these two conditions may be difficult in the clinical setting. Which of the following statements is true?

   A. Undifferentiated somatoform disorder requires the presence of persistent physical complaints for at least 12 months.
   B. Patients with chronic pain rarely also qualify for a diagnosis of undifferentiated somatoform disorder.
   C. The psychological preoccupation in hypochondriasis relates to the symptoms experienced, rather than the possible disease "represented" by the symptoms.
   D. It has been clearly established that high educational level and high socioeconomic status lead to a predisposition to hypochondriasis, because individuals with these factors may be more aware of medical conditions and have greater access to information.
   E. Comorbid depressive and anxiety disorders are common in hypochondriasis.

The correct response is option E.

Comorbid psychiatric disorders, especially major depression, panic disorder, and obsessive-compulsive disorder, are common in hypochondriasis.

Undifferentiated somatoform disorder requires the presence of persistent physical pain for at least 6 months. Patients with chronic pain have been found to have quite high rates of undifferentiated somatoform disorder. Hypochondriasis is characterized by a preoccupation with fears of having a serious illness. There is some debate regarding whether factors such as low education level, low socioeconomic status, and old age increase the risk of hypochondriasis. **(pp. 296–297)**

17.3 Conversion disorder is characterized by motor and/or sensory deficits that suggest neurological illness(es) but that cannot be elucidated by the appropriate neurological and neuroimaging evaluations. Which of the following is true regarding this syndrome?

A. Conversion disorder is more common in elderly than in young patients.

B. Conversion disorder is seen almost exclusively in women.

C. Comorbidity in conversion disorder includes substance abuse and head injury.

D. Although nonepileptic seizures (often referred to as pseudoseizures) are a subtype of conversion disorder, they are rarely seen in patients with a bona fide seizure disorder.

E. As with younger patients, elderly patients with conversion disorder infrequently have an "actual" comorbid neurological disorder.

The correct response is option C.

Comorbidity in conversion disorder includes substance abuse, chronic illness, head trauma, and previous conversion symptoms.

Conversion disorder is more common in young women, although it has also been reported in the elderly population. Nonepileptic seizures are seen in 5%–20% of outpatients with epilepsy. Conversion disorder in late life is likely associated with an actual comorbid neurological disorder. **(p. 297)**

17.4 Pain is a common complaint in geriatric medicine; therefore, appreciation of the psychiatric aspects of pain disorders is important for the physician treating these patients. Which of the following is true of pain disorders?

A. Alzheimer's disease may lower the pain threshold, thus altering the pain perception in these patients.

B. In patients with chronic low back pain, psychiatric comorbidity typically follows the onset of the chronic pain syndrome.

C. Specific descriptions of pain due solely to psychological factors can be readily distinguished from pain states where there is an "obvious" general medical condition.

D. In the Okasha et al. (1999) study on headache, somatoform pain disorder was twice as common in the nonorganic-etiology group as in the organic-etiology group.

E. In the Aigner and Bach (1999) study on chronic pain, hypochondriasis was the most common comorbid somatoform disorder.

The correct response is option D.

In the Okasha et al. 1999 study, somatoform pain disorder was diagnosed in more than 40% of individuals with no established organic etiology and in 20% of persons with an organic etiology.

Alzheimer's disease may alter pain perception by increasing the pain threshold. In a study of chronic low back pain sufferers (Polatin et al. 1993), 80% had a lifetime psychiatric illness (including major depression, substance abuse, anxiety disorders, or personality disorders) that preceded the development of chronic pain. Descriptions of pain do not differ in patients affected by pain due to psychological factors as opposed to pain due to both psychological factors and a general medical problem. In the Aigner and Bach study (1999), 90% of patients with chronic pain met criteria for undifferentiated somatoform disorder. **(pp. 297–298)**

17.5   The etiology of somatoform disorders has been subject to much theoretical speculation. Which of the following is true?

A. The prevalence of all definitively diagnosed somatoform disorders increases with age.
B. When somatoform disorders present in the older patient, comorbid neurological illness may be associated with them, but neuropsychological (cognitive) impairment is not.
C. Somatoform disorders are associated with a history of serious illness of a parent, but not in the patient, early in life.
D. Comorbid panic disorder is common in somatoform disorders, but other anxiety disorders are not.
E. The personality trait of neuroticism, wherein the subject experiences more negative emotions, is associated with the development of somatoform disorders.

The correct response is option E.

The personality trait of neuroticism is associated with the development of somatoform disorders.

The prevalence of somatoform disorders does not increase with age, with the exception of hypochondriasis. When present in late life, somatoform disorders may be associated with neuropsychological impairment and/or comorbid neurological illness. Somatoform disorders have been associated with the experience of serious illness early in life, childhood abuse, and significant psychological stress. Comorbid depression, anxiety and panic disorders, substance abuse, and personality disorders are common in somatoform disorders. **(pp. 298–299)**

17.6   Treatment of somatoform disorders calls for an integrative biopsychosocial approach by the physician. Which of the following approaches is recommended?

A. The physician should arrange appointments on an as-needed basis.
B. A focus on obtaining insight into the psychological context of somatoform symptoms should be the first priority for intervention.
C. The physician should not offer to review all prior medical records, as this merely reinforces maladaptive somatization behavior.
D. Hypochondriasis has been shown to respond to antidepressants and anxiolytics.
E. Hypnosis should be avoided in conversion disorder as these patients are rarely subject to induction of hypnosis.

The correct response is option D.

Hypochondriacal symptoms have responded to antidepressant medications, especially to selective serotonin reuptake inhibitors (SSRIs) and anxiolytics.

The physician should arrange periodic but regularly scheduled appointments and should focus on symptom reduction and rehabilitation. Offering to review all available medical records can be a tangible way for the physician to convey the seriousness given to the patient's symptoms. In conversion disorders, hypnosis is sometimes used as both a diagnostic and a therapeutic tool. **(pp. 299–300)**

References

Aigner M, Bach M: Clinical utility of DSM-IV pain disorder. Compr Psychiatry 40:353–357, 1999

Miller AR, North CS, Clouse RE, et al: The association of irritable bowel syndrome and somatization disorder. Ann Clin Psychiatry 13:25–30, 2001

Okasha A, Ismail MK, Khalil AH, et al: A psychiatric study of nonorganic chronic headache patients. Psychosomatics 40:233–238, 1999

Polatin PB, Kinney RK, Gatchel RJ, et al: Psychiatric illness and chronic low-back pain. The mind and the spine—which goes first? Spine 18:66–71, 1993

Chapter 18

Sexual Disorders

Select the single best response for each question.

18.1 Sexual function in older patients may be an important area of quality of life and needs thoughtful and sensitive clinical assessment. Which of the following statements is true regarding the Jacoby (1999) study of late-life sexuality?

A. The study involved face-to-face interviews.
B. Subjects ranged in age from 55 to 80.
C. Among respondents over age 75, men were three times as likely as women to have a steady sexual partner.
D. The majority of subjects of both sexes stated that sexual activity was important to their quality of life.
E. About 50% of respondents remained sexually active.

The correct response is option C.

The Jacoby (1999) study found that 58% of men and 21% of women older than 75 had steady sexual partners.
   The study used a mail survey. Subjects were age 45 or older; 60% of men and 35% of women said that sexual activity was important to their overall quality of life, and three-quarters of both men and women in the sample reported being sexually active. **(pp. 303–304)**

18.2 Masters and Johnson's groundbreaking research (1966) described the human sexual response in a four-stage model, each stage corresponding with specific psychological and/or physiological events. Which of the following stages is not included in Masters and Johnson's model?

A. Desire.
B. Excitement or arousal.
C. Plateau.
D. Orgasm.
E. Resolution.

The correct response is option A.

Desire was not included. Zilbergeld and Ellison (1980) added a fifth stage, desire, to account for a psychological and physiological component of sexuality. **(p. 304)**

18.3 Sexual function is affected by aging and is thus an issue of great interest to the geropsychiatrist. Which of the following statements is true regarding sexual function and age?

A. In men, testosterone levels decrease notably beginning at age 50.
B. Erectile dysfunction affects more than 50% of men ages 40 to 70.
C. Erectile dysfunction affects more than 95% of men over age 70.
D. Among older women, dyspareunia is common, but hypoactive sexual desire disorder is infrequent.
E. Impaired arousal due to diabetic vascular disease is an example of a secondary effect on sexual function.

The correct response is option B.

Erectile dysfunction affects more than 50% of men ages 40 to 70 and nearly 70% of men ages 70 or older.

Testosterone levels in men do not decrease appreciably until after age 70. In older women, the most common forms of sexual dysfunction include hypoactive sexual desire, inhibited orgasm, and dyspareunia. Diabetes, peripheral vascular disease, cancer, pulmonary disease, depression, stroke, dementia, Parkinson's disease, and substance abuse exert both primary and secondary effects on sexual function. **(pp. 305–308)**

18.4 Medications are a common cause of sexual dysfunction in older patients. Which of the following is *not* true regarding various compensatory strategies physicians can consider to address this problem?

A. Continue medication while tolerance to the medication develops, after which sexual function may spontaneously improve.
B. Reduce dose to a level without sexual side effects.
C. Try a drug holiday for a medication with a long half-life.
D. Simplify a complex regimen of medications.
E. Switch to an alternative medication with less risk of sexual side effects.

The correct response is option C.

For certain medications, such as antidepressants with a short half-life, a drug holiday can result in transient improvement in sexual function. **(p. 309)**

18.5 Unfortunately, antidepressant medications (particularly selective serotonin reuptake inhibitors [SSRIs]) have been associated with sexual dysfunction as a medication-induced side effect. There are several antidotes that the psychiatrist can use to address this problem. However, the subsequent loss of primary antidepressant effect is a concerning possibility. Which of the following antidotes can reverse the antidepressant effect of SSRIs?

A. Yohimbine.
B. Amantadine.
C. Cyproheptadine.
D. Bethanecol.
E. Methylphenidate.

The correct response is option C.

Cyproheptadine reverses the antidepressant effect of SSRIs. **(p. 309)**

18.6   Erectile dysfunction (ED) is the most common sexual dysfunction in male patients, and its risk increases with age. Which of the following is true regarding the genesis and management of ED?

   A. Erectile physiology is implicated in less than 50% of cases of ED.
   B. Hypogonadism with resultant testosterone deficiency should be treated with exogenous testosterone, even in cases of prostate cancer.
   C. Sildenafil (Viagra) is effective only in men with ED due to "organic" causes.
   D. Spontaneous erections (without physical stimulation) often follow dosing of sildenafil.
   E. Side effects of sildenafil include headache, flushing, gastrointestinal discomfort, and blurred vision.

The correct response is option E.

Side effects of sildenafil include headache, flushing, gastrointestinal discomfort, blurred vision, and hazardous increases in blood pressure if taken in conjunction with nitrates.

   Up to 80% of ED is caused by a problem with erectile physiology. Hypogonadism with testosterone deficiency is a cause of 5% of ED. Sildenafil is effective in men with ED due to psychological or organic factors. Spontaneous erections do not occur with sildenafil. **(pp. 310–311)**

18.7   Inappropriate sexual behavior in dementia may cause great disruption to caregivers and institutions managing care for these patients and thus requires effective intervention. Which of the following is *not* true regarding problematic sexual behavior in dementia?

   A. Inappropriate sexual behavior in dementia is seen in 25% of cases, whether patients are in the community or institutionalized.
   B. Caregivers and staff should set verbal limits and redirect sexually inappropriate behaviors of patients with dementia.
   C. Restrictive clothing may be used to minimize incidents of genital display and self-stimulation.
   D. Excess libidinal urges in dementia can be treated by SSRI or beta-blocker.
   E. Estrogen can be used to decrease sexual aggression in male patients with dementia.

The correct response is option A.

In various studies, inappropriate sexual behaviors in dementia were seen in 2%–7% of individuals with Alzheimer's disease, although these rates may be higher in institutionalized populations. **(pp. 313–315)**

References

Jacoby S: Great sex: what's age got to do with it? Modern Maturity 42W(5):41–45, 91, September/October 1999

Masters WH, Johnson VE: Human Sexual Response. Boston, MA, Little, Brown, 1966

Zilbergeld B, Ellison C: Desire discrepancies and arousal problems in sex therapy, in Principles and Practice of Sex Therapy. Edited by Leiblum S, Pervin L. New York, Guilford, 1980, pp 65–101

Chapter 19

Bereavement and Adjustment Disorders

Select the single best response for each question.

19.1 Bereavement is a common focus of clinical inquiry in geropsychiatry. The epidemiology of partner loss as a locus for bereavement has led to some conclusions that are of interest to the practicing clinician. Which of the following is true regarding widowhood and widowerhood in the United States?

A. The mean age of spousal loss is 3 years older for women than for men.
B. The mean duration of widowhood for women is twice that of widowerhood for men.
C. The rates of widowhood among persons older than 65 are much higher for Hispanic and Asian Americans than for Caucasians.
D. Among those older than 65, women are twice as likely as men (30% vs. 15%) to have lost a spouse.
E. Following the loss of a spouse, women are at a higher risk for mortality than are men.

The correct response is option B.

The mean duration of widowhood or widowerhood is approximately 14 years for women versus 7 years for men.

 The mean age of spousal loss is 69 years for men and 66 years for women. Among people age 65 or older, about 45% of women and 15% of men have lost a spouse. The rates of widowhood among people age 65 or older are similar for whites, Hispanics, and Asian Americans and are slightly higher for African Americans. After the loss of a spouse, older men are at higher risk for mortality than are women. **(pp. 319–320)**

19.2 Numerous theories of attachment have been posited and applied to the clinical problem of bereavement. Which of the following is true?

A. Bowlby's attachment theory holds that separation anxiety and pining serve to facilitate emotional withdrawal from the lost object.
B. In accordance with theories of adaptation, grief symptoms typically abate in elderly widows and widowers.
C. Bowlby (1980) found that preoccupation with the lost spouse 12 months after his or her death occurred only in a small minority of subjects.
D. The survivor who maintains abstract rather then concrete ties with the lost partner is more likely to manifest healthy adaptation to loss.
E. Survivors who maintain contact with the lost partner through special possessions of the deceased experience less psychological distress and grief-specific symptoms.

The correct response is option D.

Maintaining abstract rather than concrete ties with the deceased person is suggestive of healthy adaptation.

Bowlby's attachment theory holds that bereavement gives rise to separation anxiety and pining, which do not facilitate withdrawal from the lost object but rather reunion with it. Grief symptoms often do not abate in elderly widows and widowers. Bowlby found that at least half of his subjects were still preoccupied with their lost spouse more than 12 months after the loss. In a longitudinal study, Field et al. (1999) found that survivors who comforted themselves with special possessions of the deceased spouse experienced more psychological distress and grief-specific symptoms. **(pp. 320–321)**

19.3   Stroebe and Schut are notable for their recent work on a dual-process model of bereavement. According to this model, which of the following is considered to be a restoration-oriented rather than a loss-oriented stressor?

A. Emotional symptoms.
B. Behavioral symptoms.
C. New identity development.
D. Physiological symptoms.
E. Cognitive symptoms.

The correct response is option C.

Restoration-oriented stressors include developing new identities and learning new skills to perform tasks previously done by the deceased. Loss-oriented stressors are manifested as emotional, behavioral, physiological, and cognitive symptoms (Stroebe and Schut 1999). **(p. 322)**

19.4   An application of the dual-process model of grief is to focus on specific tasks required of the survivor. These are grouped into two categories: grief tasks and restoration tasks. All of the following challenges are considered to be grief tasks *except*

A. Acceptance of the changed world.
B. Confrontation of the loss.
C. Restructuring thoughts.
D. Restructuring memories.
E. Emotional withdrawal from the deceased without forgetting him or her.

The correct response is option A.

Acceptance of the changed world, spending time away from grieving, and developing new relationships and identities are considered restoration tasks. **(p. 322)**

19.5   Studies of ethnic and cultural differences in end-of-life and bereavement issues have revealed distinctions of clinical importance. Regarding Block's 1998 study of Latinos, particularly first- and second-generation, which of the following is *not* true?

A. Patients valued family input into treatment decisions.
B. Patients had extensive social networks.
C. Patients placed family interests above those of the self.
D. Patients resisted accepting death as unavoidable.
E. Patients preferred a caring rather than a scientific approach by the physician.

The correct response is option D.

First- and second-generation Latinos accept death as unavoidable, value familial input when making treatment decisions, possess extensive social networks, place family interests before self-interest, and prefer a caring, personal approach to a scientific one in the treatment process (Block 1998). **(p. 324)**

19.6   In clinical classification of cases that present with depressive symptoms in the context of interpersonal loss or grief, the physician often faces the task of deciding when symptoms cross the threshold of becoming complicated bereavement. This distinction is not always simple. To address this, DSM-IV-TR includes several specific symptoms that are not considered to be characteristic of a "normal" grief reaction. Which of the following symptoms would *not* be considered evidence of complicated bereavement?

A. Guilt about actions not taken at the time of death.
B. Preoccupation with personal worthlessness.
C. Marked psychomotor retardation.
D. Prolonged and marked functional impairment.
E. Hallucinations not containing imagery of the dead person.

The correct response is option A.

Guilt about actions not taken by the survivor at the time of death would not be considered evidence of complicated bereavement. **(p. 325)**

19.7   Several longitudinal studies of late-life bereavement have revealed some specific findings. Which of the following is true?

A. Symptoms of anxiety and depression among bereaved subjects differ from controls only in the first 2 months following the loss.
B. All studies have shown a higher psychological symptom burden among bereaved men than among bereaved women.
C. When separated operationally from other symptoms such as anxiety and depression, grief has been found to remain for longer time periods.
D. Women have been found to have higher rates of persistent grief than men.
E. Older women who have lost their spouses have a higher risk of death than older bereaved men.

The correct response is option C.

The level of grief remains high over at least a 30-month interval after a spouse's death, and the experience of grief is distinct from the experience of depressed mood and related symptoms, which lessen significantly over that same interval.

Symptoms of anxiety and depression among bereaved subjects and nonbereaved controls differ significantly in the first 2–6 months after a spouse's death. Although, typically, bereaved women report more psychological distress than bereaved men, no gender differences have been found in the level of grief reported by individuals. Older bereaved men who have lost their spouses are at higher risk for death than bereaved women. **(pp. 326–327)**

19.8 Which of the following is true regarding clinical interventions for complicated bereavement in older patients?

    A. If depression is present, it should not be treated (specifically with medications) until the grieving process is addressed.

    B. Even if major depression is present, it should not be treated for at least 4 months.

    C. Since most deaths of elderly patients are due to chronic illness, posttraumatic stress disorder in survivors is rare.

    D. Combined pharmacological and psychotherapeutic treatment has been shown to be more effective than either intervention alone.

    E. The late-life depression research group in Pittsburgh (M.D. Miller et al. 1997; Reynolds et al. 1999), used fluoxetine as its antidepressant in research studies.

The correct response is option D.

Pharmacological treatments combined with psychotherapy have been shown to be more effective than either intervention alone. If a clinical level of depression is present, it should be treated first, as early as 2 months after the loss. Posttraumatic stress disorder is also a common complication. The late-life depression study in Pittsburgh, Pennsylvania (M.D. Miller et al. 1997; Reynolds et al. 1999) used nortriptyline as the antidepressant. **(pp. 329–330)**

References

Block JB: The meaning of death, in Healing Latinos: The Art of Cultural Competence in Medicine. Edited by Hayes-Bautista D, Chiprut R. Los Angeles, CA, Cedars-Sinai Health System, 1998, pp 79–85

Bowlby J: Attachment and Loss, Vol 3: Loss: Sadness and Depression. London, Hogarth Press, 1980

Field NP, Nichols C, Holen A, et al: The relation of continuing attachment to adjustment in conjugal bereavement. J Consult Clin Psychol 67:212–218, 1999

Miller MD, Wolfson L, Frank E, et al: Using interpersonal psychotherapy (IPT) in a combined psychotherapy/medication research protocol with depressed elders: a descriptive report with case vignettes. J Psychother Pract Res 7:47–55, 1997

Reynolds CF 3rd, Miller MD, Pasternak RE, et al: Treatment of bereavement-related major depressive episodes in later life: a controlled study of acute and continuation treatment with nortriptyline and interpersonal psychotherapy. Am J Psychiatry 156:202–208, 1999

Stroebe M, Schut H: The dual process model of coping with bereavement: rationale and description. Death Stud 23:197–224, 1999

Chapter 20

Sleep and Circadian Rhythm Disorders

Select the single best response for each question.

20.1 Sleep disorders are an important and often obscure cause of clinical distress in elderly patients. As such, their full evaluation and thoughtful management may enhance patients' quality of life substantially. Which of the following is true?

A. One-quarter of noninstitutionalized persons older than 65 report chronic sleep problems.
B. Despite clinical distress due to sleep disorders, they are an infrequent reason for long-term care placement.
C. Most age-related sleep disturbances are caused by primary, as opposed to secondary, sleep-related symptoms.
D. Sleep and circadian rhythm changes in elderly patients are absent unless there is a sleep disorder.
E. With increasing age, an increased number of arousals is causative in the increased amount of nocturnal wake time.

The correct response is option E.

With increasing age, nocturnal sleep time steadily decreases and nocturnal wake time increases because of an increase in arousals.

More than half of noninstitutionalized individuals age 65 or older report chronic sleep difficulties. Sleep disturbances are among the leading reasons for long-term care placement. Most age-related sleep changes stem from an increased incidence of sleep disturbances that lead to secondary sleep-related symptoms. Changes in sleep and circadian rhythms also occur in healthy elderly individuals. **(pp. 339–340)**

20.2 Sleep apnea (SA), periodic limb movement disorder (PLMD), and restless legs syndrome (RLS) are relatively commonly encountered in older patients. Which of the following is true?

A. The more common form of SA in elderly patients is central rather than obstructive.
B. SA, even in mild cases, is not associated with insomnia.
C. The primary treatment of obstructive SA is surgical.
D. Clinically significant PLMD is five to six times more common in elderly patients, when compared to younger adults.
E. Polysomnography is required for the diagnosis of both PLMD and RLS.

The correct response is option D.

Clinically significant PLMD is seen in 30%–45% of adults age 60 years or older, compared to 5%–6% of all adults.

The predominant type of sleep apnea seen in elderly individuals is obstructive (the oropharynx collapses during attempts to breathe). Apnea generally causes excessive sleepiness, although mild to moderate apnea can be associated with insomnia. The primary treatment of obstructive SA is continuous positive airway pressure. Polysomnography is not needed for a diagnosis of RLS. **(pp. 340–341)**

20.3 Alzheimer's disease and Parkinson's disease are associated with many neuropsychiatric complications. Among these is disturbed sleep; when sleep disturbance is associated with behavioral agitation, the term "sundowning" is used. Which of the following is true regarding sleep disorders and their management in these neurodegenerative conditions?

A. Alzheimer's disease patients have increased arousals and awakenings, and increased amounts of REM and slow-wave sleep.
B. Benzodiazepines are the treatment of choice for the sundowning in Alzheimer's disease.
C. Antipsychotics may be helpful for the treatment of Alzheimer's disease patients with sundowning, and the atypical agents are generally well tolerated.
D. Sleep complaints are notable in less than one-half of Parkinson's disease patients.
E. Although carbidopa/levodopa combinations may cause initial insomnia, they do not increase risk of nightmares.

The correct response is option C.

Of all medications prescribed for sundowning, antipsychotics have the most evidence of efficacy.
    Individuals with Alzheimer's disease have increased arousals and awakenings and a diminished amount of REM and slow-wave sleep. Benzodiazepines are ineffective in the treatment of sundowning in Alzheimer's disease. Sleep complaints are noted in 60%–90% of individuals with Parkinson's disease. Carbidopa/levodopa may cause initial insomnia and cause nightmares. **(pp. 342–343)**

20.4 Comorbid medical conditions are common in older patients with sleep complaints, and the management of the chronic illness may be of great utility in assisting these patients. Which of the following is true for those patients with chronic obstructive pulmonary disease (COPD)?

A. In COPD, the degree of sleep disruption is correlated with the degree of hypoxemia.
B. Daytime sleepiness is typical in COPD.
C. Polysomnography is routinely necessary to evaluate sleep complaints in COPD because sleep apnea is much more common in these patients.
D. Oral theophyllines are adenosine receptor antagonists and may themselves disrupt sleep in COPD.
E. Benzodiazepines are the treatment of choice for COPD patients with sleep complaints.

The correct response is option D.

Oral theophyllines may have a sleep-disruptive effect in COPD treatment.
    In COPD, the degree of sleep disruption is unrelated to hypoxemia. Daytime sleepiness does not appear in COPD. Polysomnography is not routinely indicated for individuals with COPD with sleep difficulties. Sleep apnea is not more common in persons with COPD than in the general population. Benzodiazepines should be used with great caution because they may worsen nocturnal hypoxemia in COPD patients. **(p. 343)**

20.5   There are various methods by which to evaluate and classify sleep disorders. The patient who is suspected of having narcolepsy requires which of the following?

   A. Polysomnography and multiple sleep latency test (MSLT).
   B. Polysomnography and sleep log.
   C. Actigraphy and sleep log.
   D. Sleep log and MSLT.
   E. Polysomnography and actigraphy.

The correct response is option A.

An individual suspected of having narcolepsy requires polysomnography followed by an MSLT the next day. **(p. 345)**

20.6   Which of the following is true regarding treatment of sleep disorders?

   A. The majority of sleep complaints are due to a primary sleep disorder, not an associated medical condition.
   B. In patients with primary insomnia, medications are the first treatment option.
   C. The most commonly prescribed hypnotic agents are atypical benzodiazepines.
   D. Trazodone is FDA-approved for the short-term treatment of insomnia.
   E. Zolpidem has the shortest half-life of the atypical benzodiazepines.

The correct response is option C.

The most commonly prescribed medications for the treatment of sleep disorders are the atypical benzodiazepines.

   The majority of sleep complaints are due to an underlying medical or psychiatric condition. The first treatment option for patients with primary insomnia is behavioral treatment. The antidepressant trazodone is not FDA-approved for the treatment of insomnia. Zaleplon has the shortest half-life of the atypical benzodiazepines. **(pp. 346–348)**

C h a p t e r   2 1

Alcohol and Drug Problems

Select the single best response for each question.

21.1 Substance abuse and dependence problems may cause significant distress for the older patient and need to be evaluated fully by the geropsychiatrist. Which of the following is true regarding substance use disorders in this population?

   A. The prevalence of substance use disorders in patients over 65 is roughly twice as high for men as for women.
   B. Risk factors for elder substance abuse are similar to those for younger adults (e.g., male gender, lower educational attainment, and comorbid mood disorder).
   C. Because alcohol is distributed to fatty tissues, older patients' higher body fat levels cause higher blood alcohol levels.
   D. A major cause of greater psychoactive effects of alcohol on older patients is the age-related steady decrease in activity of alcohol dehydrogenase.
   E. Alcohol leads to decreased sexual drive and impotence in male patients by an antiandrogen effect.

The correct response is option B.

The risk factors for alcohol abuse in the elderly are similar to those for the general population.

   The prevalence of substance use disorder in patients over 65 ranges from 1.9% to 4.6% for men and from 0.1% to 0.7% for women. Alcohol is not distributed to fatty tissues; consequently, although older adults have higher body fat, they have higher blood levels of alcohol because of the decrease in total body water per unit mass. There is no evidence that the activity of the alcohol dehydrogenase enzyme decreases as a function of aging. Alcohol leads to decreased sexual interest and impotence due to the decrease in release of luteinizing hormone from the anterior pituitary. **(pp. 351–354)**

21.2 The physician may be consulted to manage some of the chronic effects of alcohol on neurophysiology and cognitive function in the elderly patient. Which of the following is true regarding alcohol's chronic effects?

   A. Peripheral neuropathy in alcoholics, which often follows deficiency states of thiamine and other B-complex vitamins, is seen in 25% of chronic alcoholics.
   B. The cognitive effects of alcohol typically result in a decreased overall level of intelligence as reflected in the IQ on formal testing.
   C. Focal cognitive deficits with chronic alcoholism include deficits in visuospatial analysis and nonverbal abstraction.
   D. End-stage alcoholic dementia features anterograde, but not retrograde, amnesia.
   E. Alcoholic dementia deficits are permanent; abstinence does not reverse deficits in short-term memory.

The correct response is option C.

The most common deficits in alcoholics include visuospatial analysis, tactual spatial analysis, nonverbal abstraction, and set flexibility.

Peripheral neuropathy may occur in as many as 45% of chronic alcoholic patients. Although specific clusters of cognitive functions are affected in the older alcoholic patient, intelligence remains relatively unaffected. End-stage alcoholic dementia features severe anterograde and retrograde amnesia. Patients with alcoholic dementia who abstain may exhibit stable or improved short-term memory. **(pp. 354–355)**

21.3   Regarding the use of adjunctive medications to encourage abstinence and to facilitate recovery from alcohol dependence in elderly patents, which of the following is *not* true?

A. Disulfiram may be used, with due caution, in elderly patients.
B. Naltrexone is generally well tolerated in older patients.
C. The patient should be empowered to self-administer adjunctive medication.
D. Family members should be taught to lower their threshold for concern over even nondisruptive drinking by the patient.
E. Patients have been shown to increase compliance with treatment if family members are actively involved in treatment.

The correct response is option C.

A family member should have the responsibility for administering the daily dose of disulfiram to the patient.

There is no evidence that disulfiram is contraindicated in the elderly. Atkinson et al. (1993) found that married older alcoholics were more likely to comply with treatment if their spouses also became involved in the treatment process. **(pp. 359–360)**

21.4   Abuse of or dependence on prescription medications is another common clinical problem in geriatric medicine. Which of the following is true?

A. Benzodiazepines represent approximately 20% of all medications prescribed for patients over 65.
B. Older women are twice as likely as older men to regularly use psychoactive drugs.
C. Older adults rarely share or swap prescribed medications with each other without telling their physicians.
D. Over-the-counter remedies are used nearly as frequently as prescribed medications by older patients.
E. In elderly patients, signs of lithium carbonate toxicity are unlikely if the serum level is below 1.0 mEq/L.

The correct response is option A.

Benzodiazepines represent between 17% and 23% of all medications prescribed for older adults.

About 20% of older women and 17% of men regularly use psychoactive drugs. The practice of sharing and swapping medications among older adults is not infrequent and may result in abuse or dependence, which is difficult to diagnose because older adults are hesitant to reveal they have obtained medications from another source. In Western societies, over-the-counter drugs are used even more often than prescription drugs. Symptoms of lithium carbonate toxicity in elderly patients may occur when serum levels are below 1.0 mEq/L. **(pp. 361–364)**

21.5   Which of the following is *not* true regarding alcohol use and older patients?

A. Alcohol use leads to increased mortality in midlife.
B. Among those who survive into old age, alcohol use continues to be associated with greater mortality.
C. Part of the reason for increased mortality in alcohol users is due to an increased risk of suicide.
D. The sleep in alcohol-dependent patients who are withdrawn from alcohol includes decreased REM sleep and increased slow-wave sleep.
E. When alcohol is used as a hypnotic, there is often a rebound awakening 4 hours into the sleep period.

The correct response is option D.

The sleep in alcohol-dependent patients who are withdrawn from alcohol includes decreased slow-wave sleep and decreased or interrupted REM sleep. **(p. 355)**

21.6   The useful mnemonic **FRAMES** (Miller and Sanchez) can be used to organize clinical interventions for substance abuse in the elderly patient. Which of the following statements is *not* part of the **FRAMES** schema?

A. **F**eedback about substance use.
B. **R**esponsibility to address the problem of substance use.
C. **A**bstinence as an early requirement.
D. **M**enu of patient options.
E. **E**mpathy for the patient's ambivalence and challenge.

The correct response is option C.

"Advice with regard to what the patient might reasonably do" is the correct statement for letter **A** in the **FRAMES** mnemonic (Miller and Sanchez 1994). (The letter **S** in the mnemonic corresponds to the following statement: "Self-efficacy of the patient to do something about the problem.") **(p. 358)**

References

Atkinson RM, Tolso RL, Turner JA: Factors affecting outpatient treatment compliance of older male problem drinkers. J Stud Alcohol 54:102–106, 1993

Miller WR, Sanchez VC: Motivating young adults for treatment and lifestyle change, in Alcohol Use and Misuse by Young Adults. Edited by Howard GS, Nathan PE. South Bend, IN, University of Notre Dame Press, 1994

Chapter 22

Personality Disorders

Select the single best response for each question.

22.1   Which of the following is true regarding personality disorders in older patients?

A. As research into personality disorders has increased, the phenomenon of personality disorders in the elderly has been thoroughly examined.

B. Unlike in younger patients, comorbid personality disorders in elderly patients do not appear to affect outcomes of mood disorders.

C. When an older patient's personality changes significantly due to dementia, the diagnosis is "personality change due to a general medical condition."

D. In Alzheimer's disease, the change in personality is usually an exaggeration of premorbid personality traits.

E. "Personality disorder not otherwise specified" is diagnosed rarely in elderly patients.

The correct response is option D.

In Alzheimer's disease, the change in personality is usually an exaggeration of preexisting traits.

   Although general research in personality disorders has increased, not much has been done with respect to elderly patients. Substantial evidence shows the negative effect of personality disorders on the outcome of depressive disorders. When an older patient's personality changes significantly due to dementia, the diagnosis of "personality change due to a general medical condition" does not apply. Because older patients commonly show symptoms of more than one personality disorder, the diagnosis of "personality disorder not otherwise specified" is quite common. **(pp. 369–370)**

22.2   Personality disorder diagnosis in the elderly is subject to some specific clinical and epidemiological considerations. Which of the following is true?

A. The prevalence of personality disorders in the elderly population is approximately the same as in younger patients, about 10%.

B. The prevalence of personality disorders among elderly patients with another psychiatric condition is between 25% and 65%.

C. In the older population, the association between personality and anxiety disorders is the most often reported comorbidity.

D. Cluster B personality disorders do not improve with age.

E. The association between comorbid personality disorder and mood disorder is stronger for late-onset than for early-onset depression.

The correct response is option B.

The prevalence of personality disorders in older patients with other psychiatric conditions is between 25% and 65%.

   The prevalence of personality disorders in older persons is generally lower by about half than that in younger persons. Cluster B personality disorders improve with age.

The association of personality disorders with depressive disorders in the elderly population is probably the single most reported comorbidity and is higher for early-onset than for late-onset depression. (pp. 370–371)

22.3   Vaillant's studies of the hierarchy of psychological defenses have been cited to explain personality function in old age. All of the following defense mechanisms are considered to be mature and thus adaptive *except*

A. Humor.
B. Altruism.
C. Repression.
D. Sublimation.
E. Suppression.

The correct response is option C.

Repression is not considered a mature defense mechanism.
   Mature defense mechanisms include humor, altruism, sublimation, anticipation, and suppression. **(p. 371)**

22.4   In the evaluation of personality disorders in the elderly patient, the physician can be assisted by several objective and semistructured instruments. Which of the following clinical assessment instruments is a semistructured interview rather than an ancillary self-report measure?

A. Millon Clinical Multiaxial Inventory—III (MCMI-III).
B. Personality Disorders Examination (PDE).
C. Personality Diagnostic Questionnaire (PDQ-IV).
D. Schedule for Nonadaptive and Adaptive Personality.
E. Wisconsin Personality Disorders Inventory.

The correct response is option B.

The Personality Disorders Examination is a semistructured interview. **(p. 372)**

22.5   Personality change due to degenerative frontal lobe disease is associated with difficulties in planning, conformity to social norms, experience of reward and punishment, and management of complex emotions. Clinically, these symptoms may bear strong resemblance to several DSM-IV-TR personality disorders. These specific behaviors may overlap with all of the following personality disorders *except*

A. Obsessive-compulsive.
B. Narcissistic.
C. Antisocial.
D. Borderline.
E. Paranoid.

The correct response is option A.

Personality changes due to degenerative frontal lobe disease do not overlap with obsessive-compulsive personality disorder. **(pp. 372–373)**

Chapter 23

Agitation and Suspiciousness

Select the single best response for each question.

23.1 Which of the following is true regarding the psychotic disorder of late life referred to as late-life paraphrenia?

   A. It is the late-life recurrence of an earlier onset of schizophrenia in a patient who had been symptom-free for many years.
   B. According to Kraepelin's original description, most patients were male.
   C. Psychotic symptoms of the late-life episode typically include delusions, but hallucinations are not experienced.
   D. Patients have been reported to have simultaneous sensory deficits.
   E. Antipsychotics have been demonstrated to be effective for late-life delusional disorder.

The correct response is option D.

Patients with late-life paraphrenia may have comorbid sensory deficits.

   Late-life paraphrenia identifies psychosis that has a late age at onset. According to Kraepelin, most patients were women, usually living alone. Paranoid ideation is sometimes accompanied by hallucinations. Neuroleptics are usually the first-line treatment. **(p. 377)**

23.2 The clinical evaluation of the suspicious and/or paranoid older patient requires consideration of specific concerns about psychotic disorders in older patients. Which of the following is true?

   A. Because of schizophrenic patients' tendency to isolate and have a shorter life expectancy, chronic paranoid schizophrenia is an infrequent cause of suspiciousness in elderly patients.
   B. Elderly schizophrenic patients are best managed with medication alone, rather than comprehensive treatment models.
   C. New-onset delusions in older patients are usually bizarre in nature.
   D. Antipsychotic medication should be used in all cases of sporadic agitation related to delusions.
   E. Agitation may follow family members' challenging of the patient's delusions.

The correct response is option E.

Agitation may become an issue in the elderly when they are confronted by family or clinicians about their delusions.

   Chronic paranoid schizophrenia is a major cause of suspiciousness and agitation in elderly patients. Multimodal treatment is best in elderly schizophrenic patients. New-onset delusions in older patients are usually nonbizarre. Neuroleptic medications and behavioral interventions are best used in cases of sporadic agitation related to delusions. **(pp. 377–378)**

23.3   When the physician evaluates the older patient with suspicious and/or paranoid complaints, which of the following is *not* recommended?

A. Determine whether suspicious behavior is warranted; for example, consider the possibility of neglect or abuse.
B. Challenge the delusion to verify that it is indeed fixed in the patient's mind.
C. Obtain routine laboratory studies, including chemistry and complete blood count.
D. Consider use of neuroimaging (e.g., CT or MRI of the head).
E. Consider specialty referrals for vision and hearing examination and correction.

The correct response is option B.

Challenging the delusional patient is usually not recommended.

   Routine laboratories needed in new cases of paranoia include blood chemistry, a complete blood count, and a thyroid profile. Use of neuroimaging and examinations of vision and hearing may be indicated to identify potential areas for intervention. **(p. 378)**

23.4   Agitation in dementia is a common clinical problem, for both the patient and the family. Which of the following is true regarding behavioral approaches to agitation in dementia?

A. Pharmacological approaches should precede nonpharmacological ones.
B. Patients with dementia are more likely to act out frustration with strangers than with family members because strangers are unfamiliar.
C. Agitation often correlates with other areas of impulsive behavior.
D. Because of their cognitive impairments, patients with dementia are usually nonresponsive to nonverbal behavior of caretakers.
E. Excessively calm, familiar surroundings and predictable routines unnecessarily understimulate the patient with dementia and thus should be avoided.

The correct response is option C.

Agitation is often accompanied by a loss of impulse control.

   Nonpharmacological strategies are recommended as a first-line approach. Persons with dementia are more likely to take out their frustration on those closest to them while behaving appropriately with strangers. People with dementia are extremely sensitive to the nonverbal behavior of caretakers. Agitated patients with dementia usually respond well to calm, familiar settings with predictable routines. **(pp. 378–380)**

23.5   The pharmacological treatment of dementia with agitation is necessary in many cases. Which of the following is true?

A. Among antipsychotic agents, haloperidol is clearly superior at symptom control.
B. The atypical antipsychotic agents, though less likely to cause side effects, are limited in that there is no intramuscular formulation available.
C. When a patient has consistent episodes of behavioral agitation, medication should be used on an as-needed (PRN) basis.
D. The anticonvulsants carbamazepine and divalproex are also useful in dementia with agitation.
E. Selective serotonin reuptake inhibitor (SSRI) antidepressants should be used only in the context of clear mood symptoms.

The correct response is option D.

Carbamazepine and divalproex are effective in the treatment of dementia with agitation.

There is no evidence to suggest that one atypical antipsychotic agent is more effective than another. The atypical antipsychotics ziprasidone, olanzapine, and risperidone are available in injectable forms. When a patient has consistent episodes of behavioral agitation, medication should be administered on a regular basis. SSRIs are effective even in the absence of clear depressive symptoms. **(p. 382)**

23.6   Communication strategies in dementia may facilitate the patient's maintenance of behavioral control and avoidance of escalation into agitation. All of the following communication strategies are helpful *except*

A. Ensuring adequate vision and hearing correction.
B. Maintaining good eye contact and approaching the patient slowly.
C. Decreasing "clutter" in the sensory milieu (e.g., turning off noisy electronic equipment).
D. In assisting understanding, paraphrasing, rather than simply repeating, ideas that are not apparently understood.
E. Using specific names and references and avoiding pronouns and other nonspecific language devices.

The correct response is option D.

To assist understanding between patient and clinician, the clinician should speak slowly and give the patient time to respond. Words should be repeated exactly and not paraphrased. Ask questions if the patient's meaning is unclear; be patient and reassuring. **(p. 380)**

Chapter 24

Psychopharmacology

Select the single best response for each question.

24.1   Psychopharmacological treatment of late-life psychiatric illness has significantly improved clinical function and quality of life for patients. However, systemic side effects from psychotropic medications are a vexing problem in this population. Many side effects are due to anticholinergic, antihistaminic, and antiadrenergic effects. All of the following clinical problems are referable to anticholinergic effects *except*

    A. Constipation.
    B. Urinary retention.
    C. Sedation.
    D. Delirium.
    E. Cognitive dysfunction.

The correct response is option C.

Sedation is an antihistaminergic effect. **(p. 387)**

24.2   The selective serotonin reuptake inhibitors (SSRIs) have become the first-line agents in the treatment of mood disorders in older adults. Which of the following is true regarding the use of SSRIs in older patients?

    A. Due to their pharmacokinetic profiles and low risk for drug-drug interactions, sertraline and fluoxetine are the preferred SSRIs.
    B. Several controlled trials have demonstrated the effectiveness of SSRIs in anxiety disorders in elderly patients.
    C. Despite not being technically "antipsychotic," SSRIs have been shown to be efficacious in treating delusions and hallucinations in dementia.
    D. SSRIs may cause the syndrome of inappropriate secretion of antidiuretic hormone (SIADH) with hypernatremia, which may lead to delirium.
    E. SSRIs are poorly tolerated in Parkinson's disease.

The correct response is option C.

SSRIs are effective in the treatment of behavioral disturbances with dementia, including not only agitation and disinhibition but also delusions and hallucinations.

    Escitalopram, citalopram, and sertraline are the preferred SSRIs; however, their efficacy in older patients with anxiety disorders has not been proven. A rare but dangerous adverse effect in the elderly is SIADH with significant hyponatremia. SSRIs are well tolerated by most patients with Parkinson's disease. **(pp. 388–389)**

24.3   Other contemporary antidepressants may be clinically indicated in the older patient for various psychiatric symptoms. Which of the following is true?

   A. Bupropion is contraindicated in seizure disorder patients, but it is recommended for poststroke depression.
   B. Because it may energize a fatigued depressed patient, bupropion is the antidepressant of choice in psychotic depression.
   C. Venlafaxine has different pharmacokinetic properties depending on the patient's age; thus, lower doses are typically effective for older patients.
   D. The extended-release preparation of venlafaxine significantly reduces the risk for a withdrawal syndrome when treatment is interrupted or discontinued.
   E. Mirtazapine inhibits 5-HT$_2$ and 5-HT$_3$ receptors, making it an attractive choice for elderly depressed patients with severe nausea.

The correct response is option E.

Mirtazapine is the chosen SSRI for patients with severe nausea, tremor, or sexual dysfunction.
   Bupropion is contraindicated in patients with seizure disorders and in poststroke patients and should be avoided in psychotic patients because of its dopaminergic action. Higher doses of venlafaxine are required in geriatric patients. The use of extended-release venlafaxine does not seem to reduce the incidence or severity of withdrawal symptoms. **(pp. 390–393)**

24.4   Newer agents have largely supplanted the tricyclic antidepressants (TCAs). However, some TCAs may be useful for certain patients. The secondary, rather than tertiary, amine structures are associated with less side-effect burden. Which of the following TCAs is a secondary amine and thus likely to be more tolerable by older patients?

   A. Amitriptyline.
   B. Desipramine.
   C. Imipramine.
   D. Doxepin.
   E. Clomipramine.

The correct response is option B.

Desipramine, as well as nortriptyline, is a secondary amine. **(p. 393)**

24.5   The atypical antipsychotic agents have been quickly integrated into geriatric psychiatric practice, as they are in general more tolerable than the older typical agents. Which of the following is true regarding this group of antipsychotic agents?

   A. When used for drug-induced psychosis in Parkinson's disease, clozapine should be used at doses between 100 and 200 mg/day.
   B. Olanzapine has been associated with elevated glucose and lipids, but only when there is simultaneous weight gain.
   C. Because of risk of extrapyramidal symptoms in elderly patients, doses of risperidone should be limited to less than 1 mg/day.
   D. Quetiapine does not show affinity for muscarinic receptors and is a viable alternative to clozapine for drug-induced psychosis in Parkinson's disease.
   E. Ziprasidone's use in elderly patients is limited by its high degree of muscarinic receptor affinity and resultant risk of cognitive impairment.

The correct response is option D.

In patients with Parkinson's disease and drug-induced psychosis, quetiapine is a useful alternative to clozapine.

   Clozapine should be used at low doses between 12.5 and 50 mg/day. Elevated glucose and lipids with the use of olanzapine occur even in the absence of weight gain. Risperidone is efficacious and safe at low doses of 0.5–1.5 mg/day. Ziprasidone has low potential to cause cognitive impairment and minimal impact on glucose and lipid concentrations and on weight; however, its use in older patients has been limited due to the almost total lack of geriatric data and lingering concerns regarding its potential effects on cardiac conduction. **(pp. 394–397)**

24.6   Mood stabilizers may be useful in elderly patients, both for patients with long-established bipolar disorders and for behavioral acting-out in dementing illness. Which of the following is true?

   A. Because of their greater safety profile in older patients, anticonvulsants are now prescribed much more commonly than lithium for elderly bipolar patients.
   B. Older patients are subject to lithium toxicity at lower serum lithium levels than younger adults, with cognitive impairment reported at levels even lower than 1 mEq/L.
   C. Although transient increases in liver-associated enzymes are seen in approximately 10% of patients treated with valproate, similar increases in serum ammonia are more rare.
   D. Aging alone typically increases the half-life of valproate metabolism by a factor of 2 to 3.
   E. Carbamazepine is a cytochrome P450 inhibitor and thus can inhibit its own metabolism, increasing serum levels.

The correct response is option B.

Lithium neurotoxicity in the elderly has manifested with cognitive impairment with levels well below 1 mEq/L.

   Lithium is still used more commonly than anticonvulsant medication in elders with bipolar disorder. Elevations in blood ammonia levels were present in 21% of patients receiving valproate in a study conducted by Davis et al. (1994). Aging alone does not increase the half-life of valproate. Carbamazepine concentrations are increased to potential toxicity by cytochrome P450 inhibitors but decreased by cytochrome P450 inducers. **(pp. 397–399)**

24.7   Which of these cholinesterase inhibitors is notably affected by renal function and carries an FDA warning about dose titration?

   A. Tacrine.
   B. Donepezil.
   C. Rivastigmine.
   D. Galantamine.
   E. Physostigmine.

The correct response is option C.

Rivastigmine must be titrated to prevent severe vomiting. **(p. 401)**

Reference

Davis R, Peters DH, McTavish D: Valproic acid: a reappraisal of its pharmacological properties and clinical efficacy in epilepsy. Drugs 47:332–372, 1994

Chapter 25

Electroconvulsive Therapy

Select the single best response for each question.

25.1   Electroconvulsive therapy (ECT) may be a useful intervention for several geriatric psychiatric conditions. Which of the following is true regarding ECT?

 A. In recent years, studies have shown that fewer than 25% of patients receiving ECT are older than 65.

 B. It has been conclusively shown that depression in elderly patients features more severe episodes that are more resistant to medication treatment.

 C. ECT is effective in melancholic and psychotic depression, but not in nonmelancholic depression.

 D. ECT may be effective for an acute manic episode.

 E. ECT has a specifically beneficial effect on the "negative" or deficit symptoms of schizophrenia.

The correct response is option D.

A series of reports suggests that ECT has efficacy in the treatment of acute mania. ECT has been reported to achieve a response rate as high as 80%, to have efficacy equal to that of lithium, and to have a significant advantage over lithium in patients who have not responded to lithium or antipsychotic medication.

 Thompson and colleagues (1994) reported that in 1986 approximately one-third of people receiving ECT were age 65 years or older. Some evidence shows that depressive episodes in that age group tend to be relatively more severe and also more resistant to medication, although current data are not conclusive. Regarding subtypes of depression, ECT appears to be effective in both melancholic and severe nonmelancholic depression. In addition, it may be particularly effective in psychotic major depression. No evidence indicates that ECT has efficacy for the treatment of deficit or "negative" symptoms of schizophrenia. **(p. 414)**

25.2   Which of the following is true regarding the use of ECT in elderly depressed patients?

 A. Treatment response to ECT is lower in older patients.

 B. Without maintenance treatment, less than half of successfully treated major depression cases will relapse in 6 months following ECT.

 C. The relapse rate for depression following successful ECT treatment is the same whether or not the depressive episode leading to ECT was itself medication-resistant.

 D. Randomized, controlled trials have demonstrated the benefit of maintenance ECT.

 E. Maintenance pharmacotherapy is routinely recommended following a course of ECT unless prophylactic pharmacotherapy has previously failed.

The correct response is option E.

At the present time, pharmacotherapy is usually instituted after a successful course of ECT unless at least one of the following conditions exists: 1) prophylactic pharmacotherapy has failed in the past;

2) the patient is intolerant of medications; 3) the patient has a medical illness that contraindicates medication management; or 4) the patient has a preference for prophylactic ECT.

Evidence based on data from 584 subjects suggests that, if anything, the response to ECT increases with advancing age (Sackeim 1998). A recent study showed that without receiving maintenance therapy, roughly 80% of patients successfully treated with ECT for major depression will relapse within 6 months. The relapse rate appears to be even higher among those whose depression was resistant to medication before the ECT course. However, although a number of case series and retrospective reports suggest the efficacy of continuation or maintenance ECT, no controlled, randomized studies have yet been completed. **(p. 415)**

25.3   While ECT is generally considered a second- or third-line treatment for a severe episode of depression or mania, there are certain instances where an urgent need for ECT may exist. This may be the case when the patient's condition is urgently life-threatening. All of the following circumstances would be considered life-threatening *except*

   A. Extreme, constant suicidality.
   B. Malnutrition because of poor oral intake.
   C. Dehydration because of poor oral intake.
   D. Psychosis.
   E. Inability to comply with management of a critical additional medical problem.

The correct response is option D.

First-line treatment with ECT should be considered when there is an urgent need for response in a patient with major depression or mania. This situation typically occurs when the presenting condition threatens the life of the patient because of suicidality, malnutrition, dehydration, or inability to comply with treatment of a critical medical problem. **(p. 415)**

25.4   Cognitive side effects following ECT may be quite distressing and may lead to treatment modification. Which of the following is true?

   A. Anterograde amnesia usually resolves more slowly than retrograde amnesia following ECT.
   B. Because of anterograde and retrograde amnesia, patients do not report an improvement in memory following ECT, despite improvement in mood.
   C. While patients receiving lithium are more prone to cognitive side effects after ECT, preexisting cerebral disease is not a risk factor.
   D. A larger number of ECT treatments and less time between treatments increase the risk of cognitive side effects.
   E. Unilateral electrode placement increases the risk compared to bilateral placement.

The correct response is option D.

Greater risk of cognitive side effects is associated with higher stimulus intensity, larger numbers of ECT treatments, higher dosages of barbiturate anesthetic, and less time between treatments.

Anterograde amnesia typically resolves within a few weeks after the treatment course, whereas retrograde amnesia tends to resolve more slowly. Despite objective evidence that memory performance transiently decreases after ECT, some patients indicate that their memory function improves. Furthermore, some patients, including those taking lithium and medications with anticholinergic properties—as well as those with preexisting cerebral disease—appear to be at increased risk of cognitive side effects. Bilateral placement of stimulus electrodes has been repeatedly shown to increase the risk of amnesia compared with unilateral ECT. **(p. 416)**

25.5   Increased intracranial pressure at the time of ECT has led to extreme caution about applying ECT in patients with certain CNS illnesses. Despite this concern, the risk of CNS complications remains quite low. Which of the following conditions is *not* considered a space-occupying lesion in determining the advisability of ECT?

A. Normal-pressure hydrocephalus.
B. Subdural hematoma.
C. Intracranial arachnoid cyst.
D. Arteriovenous malformation.
E. CNS tumor.

The correct response is option D.

Arteriovenous malformation is not considered a space-occupying lesion.

   Patients with a space-occupying CNS lesion such as tumors, subdural hematomas, intracranial arachnoid cysts, or normal-pressure hydrocephalus have been considered at increased risk for noncardiogenic pulmonary edema, cerebral edema, brain hemorrhage, and cerebral herniation. Although once these lesions were considered an absolute contraindication to ECT, a number of reports describe successful ECT in individuals with these lesions. **(p. 417)**

25.6   At the time of ECT, certain psychoactive drugs should be temporarily discontinued to facilitate a successful treatment episode. All of the following psychotropic medications should be held at the time of ECT treatment *except*

A. Lithium.
B. Benzodiazepines.
C. Selective serotonin reuptake inhibitors (SSRIs).
D. Bupropion.
E. Clozapine.

The correct response is option C.

SSRIs do not need to be discontinued before the administration of ECT.

   Psychotropic medications that should be avoided or maintained at the lowest possible levels are 1) lithium—it may increase the risks for delirium or prolonged seizures; 2) benzodiazepines and antiepileptic drugs—their anticonvulsant properties may decrease efficacy; 3) bupropion and clozapine—they may increase the risk of prolonged seizures. **(p. 421)**

25.7   The pre-ECT evaluation is critical in determining which patient receives ECT with the highest degree of safety. All of the following should be included in the pre-ECT evaluation in every case *except*

A. Full psychiatric history and examination.
B. Formal neuropsychological assessment of cognitive status.
C. Medical history and examination.
D. Dental history and examination for loose/missing teeth.
E. Anesthetic history and airway assessment.

The correct response is option B.

The decision about whether to pursue testing of cerebral function and structure should be made on an individual basis, guided by history and examination, but is not an absolute requirement. **(pp. 419–420)**

References

Sackeim HA: The use of electroconvulsive therapy in late-life depression, in Clinical Geriatric Psychopharmacology, 3rd Edition. Edited by Salzman C. Baltimore, MD, Williams & Wilkins, 1998, pp 262–309

Thompson JW, Weiner RD, Myers CP: Use of ECT in the United States in 1975, 1980, 1986. Am J Psychiatry 151:1657–1661, 1994

Chapter 26

Diet, Nutrition, and Exercise

Select the single best response for each question.

26.1 Assessment of nutritional status in older patients is facilitated by the use of objective measures. Numerous methods of nutritional status are available. Which of the following statements is true?

A. Standard height and weight tables are reliable in elderly patients.

B. Visceral protein stores are assessed by careful measurement of midarm circumference.

C. The most widely accepted serum marker substances for protein stores are hemoglobin and ammonia.

D. Water immersion is an accurate measure of body fat stores and is generally well tolerated by the patient.

E. Although accuracy and precision are questioned, waist and hip circumference and skin-fold caliper measurements are effective clinical tools to assess nutritional status.

The correct response is option E.

Measurement of waist and hip circumferences and skin-fold measurement by the use of calipers are easily done in the office or at the bedside and remain some of the most simple and effective tools for daily clinical work, although accuracy and precision are problematic.

Standard height/weight tables, suitable for nutritional assessment in young and middle-aged individuals, are less reliable in the elderly because of reduced height associated with vertebral compression fractures, kyphosis, and spinal disc degeneration. Although skill and experience are required, somatic protein stores can be measured by recording midarm circumference to assess muscle mass. Visceral protein stores are determined by measuring serum levels of various marker substances, of which serum hemoglobin and albumin are the most widely accepted. Water immersion is very accurate, but it requires a deep pool and is not well tolerated by patients. **(pp. 427–428)**

26.2 In parallel with protein and fat stores assessment, functional assessment of immune function is important in older patients. Which of the following is true?

A. Skin tests for immune function assess beta-lymphocyte activity.

B. Fungal antigens are injected subcutaneously.

C. Antigens commonly used include *Candida* and *Trichophyton*.

D. Since many healthy people are not reactive to these antigens, false positives are a consideration.

E. Inadequate diet is not reflected in the total lymphocyte count unless the level is less than 1,000/mL.

The correct response is option C.

Intradermal injection of fungal antigens such as *Candida* or *Trichophyton*, to which virtually every healthy person is reactive, is commonly utilized.

Skin tests to ascertain T-lymphocyte activity are useful for assessing immune system function, which declines with poor nutrition. A total lymphocyte count below 1,500/mL is useful as evidence of an inadequate diet and can be quickly determined from routine blood counts. **(p. 428)**

26.3 Prescribed medications commonly used by elderly patients with chronic systemic conditions may have effects on vitamin and nutritional requirements. Which of the following is true?

  A. Trimethoprim and phenytoin increase the need for vitamins A and E and folate.
  B. Barbiturates and cholestyramine may deplete iron and B-complex vitamins, leading to need for supplementation.
  C. Neomycin and colchicine influence absorption of fat-soluble vitamins.
  D. Patients consuming a normal diet are commonly affected by medication-induced vitamin-deficiency states.
  E. Chronic atrophic gastritis has been associated with reduced absorption of nutrients, but not elevated absorption.

The correct response is option C.

Neomycin and colchicine, as well as alcohol and cholestyramine, influence absorption of fat-soluble vitamins.

Trimethoprim and phenytoin are associated with increased need for vitamins D and K and folic acid. The use of barbiturates, cholestyramine, and also aspirin calls for extra folic acid, iron, and vitamin C in the diet. Because nutrients are abundant in a normal diet, deficits induced by medication are rarely encountered. Atrophic gastritis, often clinically undetected, affects the absorption of several nutritional factors, with both reductions and elevations having been documented. **(p. 429)**

26.4 Dietary changes have been recommended as primary preventive therapy for many chronic conditions seen in elderly patients. Which of the following is true?

  A. An emphasis on fish and grains in the diet may stabilize, but not reverse, atherosclerotic lesions.
  B. Dietary factors are as significant in cancer risk as are environmental factors and smoking.
  C. The relation between obesity and pancreatic cancer has been linked to vascular disease, not insulin levels.
  D. Diets high in saturated fats have been conclusively linked to increased risk of breast, colon, and prostate cancer.
  E. A high-fiber diet has been associated with decreased risk of both diverticula and colon cancer.

The correct response is option E.

Fiber in the diet may protect against cancer by several mechanisms. It speeds transit of fecal material through the body while it binds noxious elements, thus reducing gut contact time. The relatively low incidence of colon cancer in developing countries is explained in part by the high fiber content of primitive diets.

Emphasizing fish and grains in the diet can lead to stabilization and involution of atherosclerotic lesions. Factors such as smoking or environmental pollutants and carcinogens wield a much greater influence on cancer development than does diet. High insulin secretion associated with obesity has been linked to pancreatic cancer, establishing yet another reason to maintain normal weight. Consuming diets high in saturated fat has been associated with an increased risk of colon cancer and prostate cancer, but not breast cancer. **(p. 430)**

26.5 Tertiary prevention refers to using nutritional modification to change the course of an established disease process. Which of the following is true?

A. Osteoporosis is associated with calcium deficiency; fortunately, calcium supplements are benign, with few problematic side effects.
B. In type 2 diabetes, the Western diet adversely affects the course of the illness but not its incidence.
C. Sodium restriction to decrease intravascular volume is necessary in all edematous states, including congestive heart failure and renal failure.
D. Elevated homocysteine levels increase risk for dementia; this risk can be modified by supplemental folate.
E. Cruciferous vegetables (e.g., cauliflower and broccoli) in the diet decrease stroke risk, while other fruits and vegetables do not.

The correct response is option D.

High serum homocysteine levels are a risk factor for atherosclerotic disease and dementia. Increasing the dietary intake of folic acid will reduce homocysteine levels, which may reduce the incidence of both diseases. Some individuals experience adverse consequences from consuming calcium supplements. Intestinal discomfort is common, with symptoms of bloating or stomach pain. A Western dietary pattern is associated with a substantial increase in risk for the development of type 2 diabetes, which can be prevented by changes in the lifestyle of high-risk subjects. In patients with renal failure who develop edema, sodium restriction may be harmful if it creates a reduction in vascular volume that leads to a loss of renal perfusion pressure. Increasing the consumption of fruits and vegetables will reduce the risk of stroke. Prospective studies reveal that cruciferous and green leafy vegetables, as well as citrus fruits and juices, are protective. **(p. 431)**

26.6 Exercise is an important component of overall well-being and can be neglected in the care of older patients. Which of the following is true?

A. In diabetic patients, exercise will increase the need for insulin.
B. The exercise tolerance test (ETT) should be obtained routinely in all community-based exercise programs.
C. The ETT's greatest value is its accurate prediction of future exercise-related cardiac events.
D. Obesity levels are primarily due to activity level, not diet.
E. Maintaining exercise that produces a heart rate between 60% and 70% of maximal heart rate minimizes medical risks from exercise.

The correct response is option E.

Maintaining the target intensity of 60%–70% of maximal heart rate minimizes the risks.

People with diabetes may require adjustment in their glycemic control regimen because exercise will decrease the need for insulin. Although baseline ETT data will provide a satisfying measure of progress for the participant, the tests are expensive and are rarely required for community exercise programs. The ETT has little value for predicting adverse cardiac events. Whereas weight control is facilitated by an increase in caloric consumption related to exercise, obesity is ultimately determined by food intake. **(pp. 436–437)**

Chapter 27

Individual and Group Psychotherapy

Select the single best response for each question.

27.1 Psychotherapy may be a preferred model for certain geropsychiatric conditions. Which of the following is true regarding the general issue of psychotherapy for older patients?

   A. Because of the availability of Medicare, over 50% of older patients with psychiatric illnesses receive professional mental health care, unlike younger patients for whom insurance coverage is often problematic.

   B. Descriptive research regularly shows that older patients prefer psychopharmacological treatment to psychotherapy.

   C. Part of older patients' preference for psychopharmacological therapy is because few elders are concerned about "addiction" to antidepressants.

   D. Objective research confirms that "relationship factors" account for 80% of the variance in treatment outcomes with psychotherapy.

   E. The Luborsky meta-meta-analysis concluded that many psychotherapy models are equivalent in producing therapeutic gain.

The correct response is option E.

In an attempt to reconfirm their classic box-score analysis, Luborsky and colleagues (2002) conducted a meta-meta-analysis. They concluded that all psychotherapies are essentially equivalent in their ability to produce therapeutic gain.

   It has been estimated that only 10% of older adults in need of psychiatric services actually receive professional care, and there has been minimal utilization of mental health services in this age group. Although research on attitudes toward treatment in elderly samples is not conclusive, contrary to clinical lore, growing descriptive research suggests that older adults may prefer counseling over medication treatment. Interestingly, 56% of the same sample reported that they believed antidepressant medications to be addictive, and only 4% disagreed. Therapy also typically occurs within the context of some type of interpersonal relationship. Some have argued that relationship factors account for as much as 80% of the variance in treatment outcomes; however, research has not confirmed this assertion. **(pp. 443–444)**

27.2 When conducting psychotherapy with older patients, several factors specific to this age group should be taken into close account. All of the following are true *except*

   A. Older adults rarely respond to therapeutic interventions used with younger patients.

   B. Medical illnesses or medications may exacerbate psychiatric symptoms.

   C. The clinician must work against stereotypes about elderly patients.

   D. Older adults may not easily remember troubling earlier life events.

   E. Cognitive deficits may affect the progress of psychotherapy.

The correct response is option A.

In general, older adults will respond to many of the therapeutic interventions used with younger populations.

Medical illness or problematic medicines can exacerbate symptoms of a mental disorder. The clinician should actively work against stereotypes of elderly persons as being withdrawn, rigid, lonely, dependent, or unable to learn. Older adults may have difficulty remembering troublesome events. The clinician should consider consulting family members or longtime friends. Cognitive deficits can impede learning speed and memory. **(p. 444)**

27.3 Cognitive-behavioral psychotherapy models may be considered for older patients. Which of the following is true?

    A. Behavioral activation and automatic thought modification are equally effective at preventing relapse, and there is a powerful synergistic effect when the techniques are combined.

    B. The Blumenthal et al. study (1999) showed that the medication plus exercise group improved significantly more than the exercise-only group.

    C. The Thompson et al. study (1987) showed cognitive and behavioral therapy to be superior to brief psychodynamic therapy in reducing depression symptoms.

    D. The studies by Thompson et al. (2001) and Reynolds et al. (1999) both concluded that combined medication and psychotherapy were optimal in the treatment of depression in older adults.

    E. A logistical limitation of social problem-solving therapy is that it is not adaptable to the primary care clinic.

The correct response is option D.

The 2001 study by Thompson et al. supports conclusions by Reynolds et al. (1999) that a combined medication plus psychotherapy approach may be optimal for the treatment of depression in older adults.

Recent component analysis research suggests that behavioral activation and automatic thought modification have equal effectiveness but that both components together are no more effective in preventing relapse than when used alone. In a sample of 156 adults ages 55 and older, participants were randomly assigned to supervised exercise therapy, medication (sertraline) alone, or combined exercise and medication therapy. All three groups reported significant improvements in depressive symptoms. There were no significant differences between treatment groups, suggesting that exercise training might be comparable to the use of medication in older adults. In a study comparing cognitive, behavioral, and brief psychodynamic therapy to waiting-list control subjects, Thompson and colleagues (1987) found that all of the treatment modalities led to comparable and clinically significant reductions of depression. Problem-solving therapy can be delivered in a limited space of time; thus it can be adapted to use in primary care facilities. **(pp. 445–446)**

27.4 Another useful model for psychotherapy for depressed older adults is interpersonal psychotherapy (IPT). This model is based on four components of interpersonal relationships that lead to and maintain depressive states. These four components include all of the following *except*

    A. Grief.

    B. Interpersonal disputes.

    C. Role transitions.

    D. Interpersonal deficits.

    E. Intrapsychic or psychodynamic conflict.

The correct response is option E.

Interpersonal psychotherapy (IPT) is a manualized treatment that focuses on four components that are hypothesized to lead to or maintain depression. Whatever its etiology, depression is seen to persist in a social context. Components of treatment are 1) grief (e.g., death of spouse), 2) interpersonal disputes (e.g., conflict with adult children), 3) role transitions (e.g., retirement), and 4) interpersonal deficits (e.g., lack of assertiveness skills). **(p. 446)**

27.5   Various psychotherapy models can be utilized for the management of anxiety disorders in older patients. Which of the following is true?

  A. The most frequently used and well-substantiated psychotherapy model for geriatric anxiety symptoms is cognitive-behavioral therapy (CBT).
  B. Behavioral therapy such as progressive muscle relaxation training is contraindicated for patients with cognitive impairment.
  C. CBT appears to be the best-equipped psychotherapy model for generalized anxiety disorder (GAD) in older patients.
  D. A major limitation of CBT for geriatric anxiety states is that it cannot be conducted in the primary care clinic.
  E. Elderly patients with GAD infrequently exhibit simultaneous depressive symptoms.

The correct response is option C.

CBT appears to be the best-equipped form of psychotherapy to manage the diagnostic and treatment issues that exist in older populations with GAD.

   The most frequently used and the most well-substantiated treatments for anxiety in older adults are based on behavioral therapies. Specifically, a variety of relaxation training techniques have been pilot-tested as a treatment strategy for older adults. Patients with cognitive deficits, who may have difficulty with more cognitive strategies, may benefit from purely behavioral strategies. A pilot study by Stanley and associates (2004) presents a shortened CBT protocol for use in a primary care setting. In a sample of older adults, 60% of those who met criteria for GAD also endorsed comorbid depressive episodes. **(pp. 449–450)**

27.6   Dementia is a common condition in geropsychiatry, and psychotherapy may be a valuable adjunctive treatment option in the comprehensive care of these patients. Which of the following is true?

  A. Most empirical research on psychotherapy models for dementia is based on CBT.
  B. Reality orientation therapy for dementia has been shown to improve mastery of activities of daily living in patients with dementia.
  C. Validation therapy consists of empathic efforts to reinforce dementia patients' limited abilities to communicate.
  D. Caregiver interventions should focus solely on behavior management of the patient with dementia and not on caregiver self-care.
  E. Validation therapy is clearly more effective than general increased social support in accomplishing treatment gains.

The correct response is option C.

The premise of validation therapy is that patients who experience dementia use their remaining cognitive abilities to communicate with others.

Because of the cognitive deterioration experienced, most empirical research on interventions for dementia is based on behavioral strategies. Participants in reality orientation therapy did not differ in terms of affect measures or decline in their ability to complete normal activities of daily living. Findings suggest that interventions for caregivers that combine self-care and behavioral management strategies might prove most effective. Treatment gains from validation therapy were not significantly different from those found in the social contact condition. There is no strong support for validation therapy having greater efficacy than other interventions such as social support. **(pp. 452–454)**

References

Blumenthal JA, Babyak MA, Moore KA, et al: Effects of exercise training on older patients with major depression. Arch Intern Med 159:2349–2356, 1999

Luborsky L, Rosenthal R, Diguer L, et al: The dodo bird verdict is alive and well—mostly. Clinical Psychology Science and Practice 9:2–12, 2002

Reynolds CF 3rd, Frank E, Perel JM, et al: Nortriptyline and interpersonal psychotherapy as maintenance therapies for recurrent major depression: a randomized controlled trial in patients older than 59 years. JAMA 281:39–45, 1999

Stanley MA, Diefenbach GJ, Hopko DR: Cognitive behavioral treatment for older adults with generalized anxiety disorder: a therapist manual for primary care settings. Behav Modif 28:73–117, 2004

Thompson LW, Gallagher D, Breckenridge JS: Comparative effectiveness of psychotherapies for depressed elders. J Consult Clin Psychol 55:385–390, 1987

Thompson LW, Coon DW, Gallagher-Thompson D, et al: Comparison of desipramine and cognitive/behavioral therapy in the treatment of elderly outpatients with mild-to-moderate depression. Am J Geriatr Psychiatry 9:225–240, 2001

Chapter 28

Working With the Family of the Older Adult

Select the single best response for each question.

28.1 Which of the following is true regarding care of elderly patients with dementia in the community?

A. Fifty percent of older patients with moderate or severe dementia live alone with some level of supervision.

B. Spousal caregiver strain from care for patients with dementia is associated with increased risk of premature death.

C. Anxiety symptoms are the most commonly reported psychiatric symptoms in caregivers of patients with dementia.

D. Dependent elders are much more likely to engage in manipulative behavior than to have legitimate unmet dependency needs.

E. Defensive denial of inevitable bad outcomes in dementia must be discouraged and avoided for caregivers to give appropriate dementia care.

The correct response is option B.

Research documents that premature death is associated with spousal caregiver strain in the care of persons with Alzheimer's disease, suggesting an urgent public health preventive or protective focus for work with spouses of older adults with dementia.

Despite the high rates of shared residence, there is increasing evidence that 20% of older adults with moderate to severe dementia live alone, often with extensive supervision and assistance from local and long-distance family caregivers. Although depression is the most frequently reported psychiatric symptom among caregivers of Alzheimer's disease patients, some families express pride in their care as a legacy of commitment to family values. There is much less manipulation by dependent elders than there are real unmet dependency needs. There is more underreporting of burden and underutilization of services than the reverse. Denial is a common defense of family caregivers. Some people need to deny the inevitable outcome (loss of a beloved spouse or eventual placement of a parent in a nursing home) to provide hopeful consistent daily care. **(pp. 459–461)**

28.2 In working with dementia patients and their families, psychiatrists are advised to attend to many parallel issues in both patients and family members. All of the following are true *except*

A. Psychiatrists should monitor the mental health of caregivers as well as patients.
B. Caregivers' self-neglect and patient neglect by caregivers are both important areas for surveillance.
C. Major precipitants of the decision to place a patient with dementia in an institution are both patient factors and caregiver factors.
D. While possibly problematic, affective, anxiety, and substance abuse disorders of caregivers do not themselves predict breakdown of family care models.
E. Disruptive psychiatric symptoms by the patient with dementia strongly predict institutional placement.

The correct response is option D.

Predictors of family care breakdown are affective, substance abuse, or anxiety disorders of the primary caregiver and unresolved family conflict, all of which are amenable to psychiatric treatment of families of older adults.

Psychiatrists working with family caregivers over time will monitor the quality of family care; the mental health, capacity, and vulnerability of caregivers; and the impact of the demands of care on family relationships. Psychiatrists should be especially alert to escalating anxiety, self-neglect, suicidal ideation, depression, or anger in caregivers and abuse or neglect of the patient. Major precipitants of placement include both patient and caregiver factors. One of the patient factors that strongly predicts placement is disruptive psychiatric and behavioral symptoms. Changes in behavior and personality are also major causes of caregiver burden and depression. **(pp. 461–462)**

28.3 The conduct of office visits with dementia patients and family caregivers calls for the psychiatrist to make certain commonsense changes to clinical routine. Which of the following is true?

A. The psychiatrist should rigorously preserve patient confidentiality and not speak to family members unless the patient is present.
B. The patient should not be accompanied to the physician's office by more than one family member as this confuses the patient and leads to excessive boundary management challenges.
C. Older couples with long relationships often prefer to face medical challenges together rather than singly.
D. Psychiatrists should not encourage family members to remove weapons from the home of patients with dementia, as this is an invasion of privacy.
E. The psychiatrist should not encourage physical activity for the patient with dementia as the patient needs to preserve energy for cognitive tasks.

The correct response is option C.

Older couples in first marriages are generally more comfortable facing threatening health information together.

Although the older adult is entitled to initial time alone with the psychiatrist, later time alone with family informants will be invaluable in assessing the impact of functional loss and other family stressors. It may be helpful to have two family members accompany the patient for an evaluation. One family member can distract or sit with the older adult while another family member has a private conversation with the psychiatrist. A family concerned about the increasingly combative behavior of an older adult male may be helped by a psychiatrist who responds, "First, let's get the guns out of the house." Increasing evidence shows that encouraging physical activity and actively assessing and treating sleep disorders in older adults and their family caregivers are associated with positive care and family outcomes. (pp. 462–464)

28.4   The psychiatrist caring for patients with dementia also needs to assess the family members of the patient. Which of the following is *not* true?

   A. Older husbands who are caregivers are at increased risk of alcohol abuse.
   B. Caregivers should be encouraged to pursue regular exercise.
   C. The caregiver has a need for social stimulation while caring for a dependent elder.
   D. Secondary family support should be assessed.
   E. The psychiatrist should not directly address the caregiver's own health, as this is a matter for that person's own physician.

The correct response is option E.

The psychiatrist should ask specifically about the primary caregiver's health.

   Older husband caregivers are particularly at risk of increased alcohol use in response to care demands. The psychiatrist should be alert for positive activities such as regular exercise, social stimulation, and secondary family support. (p. 465)

28.5   When handling diagnostic/prognostic communications and while recommending additional services to the family of patients with dementia, which of the following is true?

   A. Some Asian American families regard use of formal supportive services as a moral failure.
   B. Families rarely tolerate the demands of terminal care of an immobile and incontinent patient but can usually manage the disruptive sleep and behavior of moderate dementia.
   C. Combined interventions, while appealing, have not been shown to decrease caregiver depression.
   D. Health care decisions should not be made until the diagnosis of dementia is clear and there have been several months of follow-up to estimate rapidity of progression.
   E. Families should be advised that judgment about financial matters is usually unimpaired in early dementia.

The correct response is option A.

In some Asian American families, use of any formal services may be viewed as a moral failure of the family.

   Some families cope well with end-of-life care for an immobile or incontinent older adult but are unable to tolerate the disruptive behaviors or sleep patterns of persons with moderate dementia. Combining individual and family counseling, family education, support group participation, and sustained availability of a care manager is associated with decreased caregiver burden and depression; decreases in the elder's disruptive symptoms; and increased caregiver satisfaction, subjective well-being, and self-efficacy. Handling money and health care decisions should be addressed soon after diagnosis to ensure time for patients to select a surrogate. Families must be reminded that financial judgment is impaired early in dementia. (pp. 465–468)

28.6   Driving is often a contentious issue in dementia. Which of the following is *not* true regarding driving by cognitively impaired patients?

A. Dementia leads to decreased judgment.
B. Increased reaction time is common in dementia.
C. Patients with dementia will respect the loss of their driver's license and cease to try to drive.
D. Mechanically disabling the car reduces the need to confront the patient with his or her lost skills.
E. Families should proactively arrange for alternative transportation to decrease the incentive for the patient to try to drive.

The correct response is option C.

Anonymous reports to the department of motor vehicles may lead to required testing or removal of the patient's license, but the absence of a license rarely stops a determined older adult with dementia.

Families can be encouraged to assess driving capacity based on observations of current driving, with reminders that dementia affects judgment, reaction time, and problem solving. Shaving the patient's keys, substituting another key, removing a distributor cap, or otherwise disabling a car can sometimes reduce the need to confront the patient with lost skills. The family can also work on solutions that limit the need for driving—delivery services, senior vans, or offers of regular rides to church or for visits. **(pp. 468–469)**

Chapter 29

Clinical Psychiatry in the Nursing Home

Select the single best response for each question.

29.1   Which of the following is true in the United States according to the 1995 National Nursing Home Survey (Gabrel and Jones 2000)?

A.   Between 9% and 10% of U.S. residents over the age of 65 resided in nursing homes.
B.   Compared to an earlier survey done in 1985, the percentage of older adults residing in nursing homes had increased by 0.5%.
C.   Between 1985 and 1995, the mean age of nursing home residents had increased by 2.9 years.
D.   Over 50% of women older than 85 lived in nursing homes.
E.   Among nursing home residents over 65, over 40% had vision and hearing impairments.

The correct response is option D.

Fifty-six percent of women ages 85 years and older were living in nursing homes according to the 1995 National Nursing Home Survey (Gabrel and Jones 2000).

The number of U.S. residents over the age of 65 who resided in nursing homes was 4.13%, a decline of 0.5% in the proportion of adults residing in nursing homes. Between 1985 and 1995, the mean age of nursing home residents increased by 0.9%, with the proportion of residents ages 85 and older increasing from 49% to 56% for women and from 29% to 33% for men. **(p. 473)**

29.2   The prevalence of psychiatric disorders in nursing home residents has been the subject of several studies. Which of the following is *not* true?

A.   Interview-based studies have found prevalence rates of psychiatric illness in nursing home residents as high as 94%.
B.   The Rovner et al. study (1990) found that two-thirds of nursing home residents had dementia.
C.   The Medical Expenditures Panel Survey (MEPS) found a rate of depressive disorders in nursing home residents of 20%.
D.   The MEPS study was based on clinical interviews.
E.   Rovner et al. (1990) found a prevalence of psychiatric illness of 80% in new nursing home admissions.

The correct response is option D.

The Medical Expenditures Panel Survey (Krauss and Altman 1998) was not derived from clinical interviews.

On the basis of psychiatric interviews of subjects in randomly selected samples, investigators found prevalence rates of psychiatric disorder to be as high as 94%. The Rovner study (1990) found that 67.4% of residents had dementia. The MEPS study revealed that 70%–80% of residents had cognitive impairment and 20% had a diagnosis of depressive disorder. Rovner reported that the prevalence of psychiatric disorder among persons newly admitted to a nursing home was 80.2%. **(pp. 473–474)**

29.3   Among psychiatric illnesses in nursing home residents, disorders of cognitive impairment are of great importance. Which of the following is true?

A. Among dementia subtypes, Alzheimer's disease accounts for 75% of cases, with Lewy body dementia the second most common dementia.
B. Delirium has been found in 20% of nursing home residents, primarily due to underlying dementia.
C. Psychotic symptoms are seen in 25%–50% of dementia patients in nursing homes.
D. Most psychiatric consultations in nursing homes are for psychotic episodes.
E. Behavioral disturbance in dementia is solely due to cognitive impairment.

The correct response is option C.

Psychotic symptoms have been reported in approximately 25%–50% of residents with a primary dementing illness.

Among dementia subtypes, Alzheimer's disease accounts for about 50%–60% of cases and vascular dementia accounts for about 25%–30%, while Lewy body dementia has not been ascertained in nursing home populations. Delirium is common in nursing homes and occurs primarily in patients made more vulnerable by a dementing illness. Available studies indicated that approximately 6%–7% of residents were delirious at the time of evaluation. The majority of psychiatric consultations in long-term-care settings are for evaluation and treatment of behavioral disturbances such as pacing and wandering, verbal abusiveness, disruptive shouting, physical aggression, and resistance to necessary care. **(p. 474)**

29.4   In addition to cognitive disorders, mood disorders are common psychiatric illnesses in nursing home residents. Which of the following is true?

A. Depressive disorders are the second most common psychiatric illness in nursing home residents.
B. The rate of mood disorders in nursing home residents in the United States is substantially higher than in other industrialized nations.
C. Depression in nursing home residents increases morbidity, but not mortality, rates.
D. Because of concurrent chronic medical illnesses, the DSM-IV-TR diagnostic criteria for mood disorders are not clinically valid in nursing home residents.
E. There is a subtype of depression in nursing home residents featuring low serum albumin, high levels of psychosocial disability, and prompt response to treatment with nortriptyline.

The correct response is option A.

Depressive disorder represents the second most common psychiatric diagnosis in nursing home residents. Most studies in U.S. nursing homes show depression prevalence rates of 15%–50%.

Studies from other countries have shown similar rates. In addition to its association with morbidity, depression has been found to be associated with an increase in mortality rates. DSM-IV-TR diagnostic criteria remain valid as predictors of treatment response, since the symptoms of major depression in frail elderly patients characterize a disease similar to that which occurs among younger psychiatric patients, even though most nursing home patients have concurrent medical illnesses and disabilities that complicate diagnosis and treatment. There is evidence for a clinically relevant subtype of depression in nursing home residents that is characterized by low levels of serum albumin and high levels of self-care deficits—it is not responsive to treatment with nortriptyline. **(pp. 475–476)**

29.5   Intervention for psychiatric illnesses in nursing home residents is a major clinical focus of the geropsychiatrist. Which of the following is true?

A. A program of daytime physical activity and nursing interventions to promote nighttime sleep may decrease depression, but not agitation.

B. Outcome studies on psychotherapy models in nursing home residents are derived from illness-specific interventions.

C. Risperidone has been shown to have a beneficial effect on psychotic symptoms but not independent effects on agitation or aggression.

D. Risperidone has been repeatedly demonstrated to have beneficial long-term effects on psychosis in nursing home residents.

E. The majority of nursing home residents who are withdrawn from antipsychotic agents do not experience a reemergence of psychosis.

The correct response is option E.

The majority of patients who had been receiving long-term treatment with antipsychotic agents could be withdrawn from these agents without reemergence of psychosis or agitated behaviors.

Reductions in agitation were observed in a study of a daytime physical activity intervention combined with a nighttime program to decrease noise and sleep-disruptive nursing care practices. Patients in most outcome studies were not selected on the basis of specific psychiatric symptoms or syndromes, but rather on the basis of age, cognitive status, or mobility. Risperidone has been shown to have antipsychotic effects and also independent effects on agitation or aggression. **(p. 480)**

29.6   Several concerns noted in the 1970s and 1980s in the United States led to various legal and regulatory initiatives to improve the psychiatric care in nursing homes. Which of the following is true?

A. A 1977 survey in the United States revealed that 10% of nursing home residents were physically restrained.

B. Mechanical restraints independently decrease physical agitation.

C. Nursing home patients with nonpsychotic causes of agitation nonetheless require antipsychotic medications.

D. The 1986 Institute of Medicine report found that antipsychotic drugs were being overused in nursing homes.

E. The 1986 Institute of Medicine report found that antidepressant drugs were being overused in nursing homes.

The correct response is option D.

The 1986 Institute of Medicine report highlighted problems in the overuse of antipsychotic drugs and the underuse of antidepressants for the treatment of affective disorders.

A 1977 U.S. survey of nursing home residents showed that 25% were restrained by geriatric chairs, cuffs, belts, or similar devices, primarily to control behavioral symptoms (National Center for Health Statistics 1979). Mechanical restraints have often been used in attempts to control agitation, but they do not, in fact, decrease behavioral disturbances. Patients with nonpsychotic behavioral problems may be more appropriately managed with medications other than antipsychotics. **(pp. 485–486)**

29.7   In the United States, federal regulation has led to modified practices in nursing homes. Which of the following is true?

  A. An initial first-stage screening looking for mental disorders in nursing home admissions specifically includes dementia.
  B. The second-stage assessment requires a psychiatric evaluation.
  C. Patients with dementia are required to have both a psychiatric and a neurological evaluation.
  D. The Minimum Data Set (MDS) must be administered only once to a nursing home resident.
  E. Resident Assessment Protocols (RAPs) are solely for monitoring of the use of psychotropic medication.

The correct response is option B.

The second-stage assessment requires a psychiatric evaluation to ascertain whether the patient has a mental disorder, to make a psychiatric diagnosis, and to determine whether there is a need for acute psychiatric care that precludes adequate or appropriate treatment in a nursing home.
  The initial first-stage assessment excludes dementia. Patients found to have dementia on the first screening are exempt from the preadmission psychiatric evaluation. MDS must be administered on a regular basis by members of an interdisciplinary health care team. RAPs are designed to 1) help nursing home staff recognize symptoms that are indicators of clinically significant problems, 2) conduct evaluations that use standardized algorithms, and 3) determine the need to alter the treatment plan. **(pp. 486–487)**

29.8   Concern had been raised about the use of "unnecessary drugs" in psychiatrically ill nursing home patients. All of the following constitute an "unnecessary drug" use *except*

  A. Drug used at an excessive dose.
  B. Drug used for excessive duration.
  C. Drug used with inadequate monitoring.
  D. Drug used despite adverse consequences.
  E. Drug used for other than FDA-approved indications ("off-label").

The correct response is option E.

"Unnecessary drugs" are described as any drug used in excessive dose, for excessive duration, without adequate monitoring, or in the presence of adverse consequences. Physicians may prescribe off-label medication if the clinical rationale is clearly documented in the medical record. **(p. 487)**

References

Gabrel C, Jones A: The National Nursing Home Survey: 1995 Summary. Vital Health Stat 13(146):1–83, 2000

Institute of Medicine, Committee on Nursing Home Regulation: Improving the Quality of Care in Nursing Homes. Washington, DC, National Academy Press, 1986

Krauss NA, Altman BM: Characteristics of Nursing Home Residents—1996. MEPS Research Findings No 5 (AHCPR Publ No 99-0006). Rockville, MD, Agency for Health Care Policy and Research, 1998

National Center for Health Statistics: The National Nursing Home Survey (DHEW Publ No PHS-79-1794). Hyattsville, MD, National Center for Health Statistics, 1979

Rovner BW, German PS, Broadhead J, et al: The prevalence and management of dementia and other psychiatric disorders in nursing homes. Int Psychogeriatr 2:13–24, 1990

Chapter 30

The Continuum of Care: Movement Toward the Community

Select the single best response for each question.

30.1 The trends toward community-based care rather than institutionally based care have been subject to many demographic and epidemiological variables as well as policy and programmatic considerations. Which of the following is true?

A. Primarily due to the burgeoning of the elderly population living longer with chronic illness, disability in the U.S. population has been increasing at the rate of 2% per year for the past several decades.

B. Between 1983 and 2003, the occupancy rate at available nursing homes has increased steadily.

C. Medicare devotes a large percentage of its resources to long-term care.

D. Community-based care for chronically impaired adults is lower cost than institutional care.

E. Recent initiatives for long-term care models come not from federal initiatives but from a series of organizations such as professional and community organizations.

The correct response is option E.

The new dynamic does not flow primarily from federal policy initiatives but reflects pragmatic private initiatives of professional organizations such as the Institute of Medicine, population change, and state and community initiatives for housing and caring for frail and disabled persons.

Recent confirming evidence indicates that disability in the U.S. population has apparently been declining at a rate of about 1% a year over the past several decades. Furthermore, since 1983, the occupancy rate of available nursing home beds has continued to decline. There has never been any provision for Medicare to underwrite long-term care beyond limited posthospitalization care, most often provided initially in nursing homes. Compared with nursing home care, serving high-need chronically impaired persons in the community costs more—and paradoxically, the cost of community care can seem deceptively low because it is substantially provided not by public dollars but by private family resources. **(pp. 501–502)**

30.2 The set of specific judgments by individuals that they can perform competently and capably in specific situations is referred to as

A. Self-esteem.

B. Self-efficacy.

C. Collective efficacy.

D. Actualization.

E. Ego integrity.

The correct response is option B.

Self-efficacy refers to specific judgments by individuals that they can perform competently and capably in given situations. An important extrapolation of self-efficacy is provided by the concept *collective efficacy*, which has been usefully applied in social survey research to identify collectivities such as neighborhood and community characterized by a shared sense of trust and the reliable availability of help. **(p. 503)**

30.3   The movement toward hospice care for terminally ill patients has been a major innovation in community-based care. Which of the following is *not* true regarding hospice care?

    A.   In both England and the United States, hospice emphasizes home care rather than institutional care.

    B.   A major emphasis in hospice care is adequacy of pain management.

    C.   Hospice care in the United States is covered by Medicare.

    D.   Hospice care at end of life reduces costs.

    E.   Hospice care is an appropriate model for both cancer and AIDS patients.

The correct response is option A.

Whereas the English hospice was a community of caring for the dying within institutional walls, the American version has emphasized home care, or "hospice without walls."

    The philosophy emphasizes the importance of a homelike environment for terminal care, effective pain control, the absence of high-technology medical and surgical interventions characteristic of hospitals, and emotional support for dying patients and their families. This strategy of terminal care, covered by Medicare since the mid-1980s, does tend to reduce cost of care at the end of life. Hospice, in sum, has become a major community alternative for terminal care—particularly for patients with cancer, and more recently for those with AIDS. **(p. 504)**

30.4   Assisted living models may be a useful alternative care plan for many elderly patients with support needs. Which of the following is true?

    A.   In the United States, older patients are more likely to be in substandard housing than adults of all other age groups.

    B.   The majority of older adults in the United States live alone.

    C.   Assisted living housing includes a private, self-contained personal living space.

    D.   Responsibility for care is solely limited to patients and families.

    E.   Assisted living is a low-cost option for frail elders, with few economic barriers to access to this model.

The correct response is option C.

The four concepts of the philosophy of assisted living housing in its ideal form are 1) offering a private, self-contained space of one's own; 2) matching reliably available services with measured individual need; 3) sharing responsibility for care among residents, family, and staff; and 4) making information available to residents to promote informed choices and control of their lives.

    Studies of housing and living arrangements in the United States indicate that, overall, older persons are among the best-housed adults in a well-housed nation. Only a minority of older adults (though a significant minority) live alone. Affordability is clearly a problem of the new housing option: the average annual income of current residents is $31,000. **(pp. 505–506)**

30.5   An easily neglected problem is housing and support for chronic mentally ill patients who have grown old. Which of the following is true?

A. The broadening of mental health programs in the 1970s specifically addressed the mental health needs of older patients.
B. Mental health "carve-outs" control costs solely by limiting psychiatric hospital utilization.
C. In the United States, the Older Americans Act specifically addresses the mental health needs of the elderly.
D. In the United States, federal funding through the Administration on Aging mandates specific mental health program funding at the community level.
E. Because of the existence of clear federal policies on mental health care of older patients, this issue is not considered a state or local responsibility.

The correct response is option C.

The Older Americans Act specifically discusses mental health needs; however, federal funding in support of this legislation through the Administration on Aging has not included specific mandates for mental health funding.

  In the mid-1970s mental health services were broadened to include special populations such as mentally retarded and developmentally delayed persons and those with substance abuse problems, not elders. Mental health services for older adults were rarely featured in community programs. One symptom of the current interest in cost control of mental health services is the practice of the "carve-out" of such services from managed care insurance. This practice refers to contracting with behavioral health companies specifically to provide reduced cost by limiting the number of services provided and the number of hospital days allowed. In the absence of a cohesive federal policy, responsibility for community care has largely fallen on the state, with mixed results. **(pp. 507–508)**

30.6   The Robert Wood Johnson Foundation's Community Partnership for Older Adults program was established in 2001 to enhance community care models. Which of the following is *not* true regarding this initiative?

A. Blends collaborative community partnerships and knowledgeable consumers.
B. Mobilizes community to create awareness of contributions and needs of older citizens.
C. Educates consumers to become more informed.
D. Promotes better quality of care and quality of life within existing and new programs.
E. Leverages solely private financial resources to meet identified community needs.

The correct response is option E.

This national program is based on the powerful melding of the collective efficacy of collaborative community partnerships and the self-efficacy of knowledgeable consumers. The program's goals are 1) to mobilize the community to create greater awareness of the unique contributions and increasing needs of older community members, 2) to educate community members to be more knowledgeable consumers and more effective decision makers, 3) to promote a better quality of life and care by enhancing choices and decision making by older adults and their caregivers within both existing and new programs, and 4) to leverage public and private resources in response to identified community needs so that access to care will improve. **(p. 508)**

Chapter 31

Legal, Ethical, and Policy Issues

Select the single best response for each question.

31.1 Medicare provides funding for a great deal of medical and mental health care to older patients in the United States. Which of the following is true regarding this program and mental health care?

    A. Psychotropic medication management is subject to a 50% copayment from the patient.

    B. To enhance the use of lower-cost service models, Medicare payment policies discourage acute inpatient psychiatric hospitals while encouraging outpatient psychiatric care.

    C. There is a 190-day lifetime limit for inpatient psychiatric care, which pertains to both freestanding and general hospital-based psychiatric units.

    D. Despite the benefits available in Medicare, only 6%–8% of older adults receive outpatient mental health services.

    E. Medicare Part C plans with managed care programs have become the choice of 50% of older patients.

The correct response is option D.

Despite the 14%–17% prevalence of clinically significant mental disorders among older adults residing in community settings, it is estimated that only 6%–8% of older adults actually receive outpatient mental health services.

    Medical management of psychotropic medications was exempted from this limit, and the copayment for these services was reduced to 20% under OBRA-87. Medicare payment policies for mental health care continue to encourage the use of acute inpatient services. Traditional fee-for-service Medicare Part A coverage for inpatient psychiatric hospital care sets a 190-day lifetime limit for care rendered in freestanding psychiatric hospitals but no time limit on care rendered on psychiatric units in general hospitals. Participation in Medicare Plus Choice plans declined in the late 1990s. In 2000, 16.4% of all Medicare beneficiaries were enrolled in these plans. **(pp. 515–516)**

31.2 Which of the following is *not* true regarding federal regulation of nursing homes in the United States?

    A. Regulatory concern in the 1980s focused on the inappropriate use of chemical restraints.

    B. Regulatory concern in the 1980s focused on the inappropriate use of physical restraints.

    C. In the 1980s, there was concern that antidepressants were being prescribed excessively in nursing homes.

    D. The Omnibus Budget Reconciliation Act of 1987 contained the Nursing Home Reform Act; this act addressed mental health care issues in nursing homes.

    E. Nursing home applicants must now have a preadmission assessment to establish psychiatric needs and appropriate placement.

The correct response is option C.

Regulatory focus on nursing homes was prompted in the 1980s by a combination of factors: 1) concerns about the inappropriate use of physical and chemical restraints, 2) concerns about inadequate treatment of depression (Institute of Medicine 1986), and 3) cautions from the federal Office of Management and Budget that older adults with chronic mental illness were being discharged from state mental hospitals and admitted to nursing homes, thereby shifting the cost of their care from the states to the federal government. Congress responded by passing the Nursing Home Reform Act as part of OBRA-87. The resultant HCFA regulations required preadmission assessment to identify nursing home applicants with mental illness who required acute psychiatric care and to ensure that they were appropriately placed in residential or treatment settings. (p. 517)

31.3   The Health Care Financing Administration (HCFA) in 1999 introduced 24 quality indicators for nursing homes. Quality indicators pertinent to geriatric psychiatry include all of the following *except*

   A. Behavior problems.
   B. Emotional problems.
   C. Cognitive patterns.
   D. Psychotropic drug use.
   E. Percentage of patients receiving psychiatric consultation.

The correct response is option E.

Quality indicators that pertain to geriatric mental health encompass behavior problems, emotional problems, cognitive patterns, and psychotropic drug use. **(pp. 517–518)**

31.4   Ethical issues at the end of life are an important consideration in the care of the older patient. Which of the following is *not* included in the Joint Commission on Accreditation of Healthcare Organizations core principles for end-of-life care?

   A. Respect dignity of patient and caregivers.
   B. Encompass alleviation of pain and other physical symptoms.
   C. Assess and manage psychosocial problems.
   D. Provide access to palliative and/or hospice care.
   E. Limit access to potentially harmful nonvalidated treatments, such as alternative and nontraditional treatments.

The correct response is option E.

The Joint Commission on Accreditation of Healthcare Organizations developed a list of core principles for care at the end of life: provide access to any therapy that may realistically be expected to improve the patient's quality of life, including alternative or nontraditional treatments; respect the dignity of both patient and caregivers; encompass alleviation of pain and other physical symptoms; assess and manage psychological, social, and spiritual/religious problems; and provide access to palliative care and hospice care. **(p. 520)**

31.5   Which of the following is true regarding advance directives?

   A. Patients receiving care funded by Medicare or Medicaid are required to execute advance directives.
   B. A power of attorney for health care requires notarization in all 50 U.S. states.
   C. "Durable power of attorney" is synonymous with "legal guardianship."
   D. A living will confers a wider scope of decision making than a power of attorney for health care.
   E. Compliance with advance directives by medical institutions remains poor.

The correct response is option E.

The level of compliance by the health care profession with the preferences of patients, even when these have been explicitly stated, continues to be poor.

The Patient Self-Determination Act (PSDA; 1991) requires hospitals, nursing homes, and organizations receiving Medicare and Medicaid funds from the federal government to notify patients of their right to express their wishes concerning life-sustaining care and of the laws of the relevant state with respect to advance directives. The law does not require patients to sign such a document. Advance directives for health care should include a power of attorney for health care. In some states this document requires notarization. Power of attorney differs from guardianship in that the power of attorney is given by a competent individual, whereas guardianship is imposed on one deemed incompetent. The durable power of attorney is one that survives (or comes into existence upon) the disability of the principal. The living will is generally made in association with a durable power of attorney for health care, which confers wider scope on the decision-making right. **(p. 522)**

31.6   Which of the following is true regarding legal competency for decision making?

   A. Competency can be determined by the decision of any psychiatrist.
   B. Competency can be determined by the decision of a psychiatrist, only if he or she is board-certified.
   C. Competency requires a court decision, not a medical one.
   D. Making a will and executing a power of attorney require the same level of competency.
   E. The court may request a written report but may not compel the physician to personally testify in competency cases.

The correct response is option C.

Competency requires a legal determination by a court. The standards applied in establishing competency vary with the purpose for which the evaluation is being performed. Making a will requires the lowest level of competency, whereas higher levels are required for executing a power of attorney. The court may rely on the psychiatrist's written report or may require the psychiatrist to testify in person. **(p. 524)**

Reference

Institute of Medicine, Committee on Nursing Home Regulation: Improving the Quality of Care in Nursing Homes. Washington, DC, National Academy Press, 1986

Chapter 32

The Past and Future of Geriatric Psychiatry

Select the single best response for each question.

32.1　Which is true regarding the roles of the National Institute on Aging (NIA), the National Institute of Mental Health (NIMH), Medicare, and other sponsoring agencies in geriatric psychiatry?

　　A. The NIA is the office of responsibility for research into psychiatric illnesses affecting the elderly population, for example, major depression.

　　B. The NIMH leads efforts on Alzheimer's disease research.

　　C. The NIMH is responsible for direct funding support for over 50% of geriatric psychiatric fellowships.

　　D. The Department of Veterans Affairs (VA) supports the most comprehensive system of care for mentally ill older adults in the United States.

　　E. Medicare's capitation payments system using diagnosis-related groups (DRGs) is applied to inpatient psychiatric care.

The correct response is option D.

The VA currently supports the most comprehensive system of care for mentally impaired older adults, including acute inpatient hospitalization, outpatient clinics, long-term-care facilities, and domiciliary care.

　　NIA has led the effort in Alzheimer's disease research, whereas research in other geriatric psychiatric disorders, especially major depression, has been led by NIMH. There are now a rapidly increasing number of geriatric psychiatry fellowship programs, although few currently receive NIMH support. These programs have been funded primarily through the Department of Veterans Affairs (VA), state support, and support from individual medical centers. The capitation of payments for certain illnesses via DRGs was instituted in 1983, although DRGs have yet to be applied to inpatient psychiatric disorders. **(pp. 530–532)**

32.2　Geriatric psychiatrists may practice preventive psychiatry in many instances. Which of the following interventions would be a primary prevention effort?

　　A. Provision of adequate social and logistical support to decrease loneliness and despair, preventing the onset of major psychiatric illness.

　　B. Early diagnosis of major depression and provision of supportive psychotherapy.

　　C. Early diagnosis of major depression and provision of supportive psychotherapy plus pharmacotherapy.

　　D. Early diagnosis of major depression and provision of pharmacotherapy.

　　E. Rehabilitation of patients with dementia who are managed in a long-term care facility.

The correct response is option A.

Forced isolation and the absence of effective communication with other persons contribute to the onset of major depression and paranoid psychoses. It is at this level that the geriatric psychiatrist may achieve the greatest success, given the limited resources available.

Early diagnosis of major depression permits the psychiatrist to attempt a rational course of outpatient antidepressant therapy before the complications of excess medication or neglect of physical health ensue during the course of a depressive illness. Tertiary prevention is directed toward preventing the disability that may result from mental illness. Rehabilitation techniques are important in long-term care facilities, especially in the management of care for patients with dementia. **(p. 533)**

32.3 The concept of "successful aging" is associated with the concept of "wisdom" as articulated by Baltes (1993). Which of the following is *not* included under the components of wisdom as described by Baltes?

A. Factual knowledge.
B. Procedural knowledge.
C. Life-span contextualization.
D. Value absolutism.
E. Acceptance of uncertainty.

The correct response is option D.

Baltes (1993) emphasized the importance of wisdom in successful aging, something that cannot be measured quantitatively. For example, he suggested that wisdom includes 1) factual knowledge (the data necessary to respond to a situation); 2) procedural knowledge (strategies of acquiring data, making decisions, and providing advice); 3) life-span contextualization (recognizing the inner relationships, tensions, and priorities of different life domains within the context of the life span); 4) value relativism (ability to separate one's own values from those of others); and 5) acceptance of uncertainty (recognizing that no perfect solution exists and optimizing the resolution of a situation as well as possible). **(p. 534)**

32.4 Which is true regarding the subspecialty board certification in geriatric psychiatry in the United States?

A. The first examination was given in 1981.
B. Applicants must now complete a 1-year fellowship in geriatric psychiatry to take the examination.
C. Certifications are for 5 years.
D. Recertifying examinations are closed-book format.
E. The added credential is officially called "Added Qualifications in Geriatric Psychiatry."

The correct response is option B.

Only 83 certificates were issued in 2000—primarily because of the newer requirement that all psychiatrists who sit for the examination must have completed a 1-year fellowship in geriatric psychiatry, in contrast to the "grandfather clause" used for the first two examinations and certifications.

The first examination was given in 1991; more than 800 persons sat for the examination, and more than 500 passed it. The original certification was for 10 years, and the first recertifying examination was given in 1991—an open-book examination, in contrast to the original closed-book examination. The added credential is now called "Certification in the Subspecialty of Geriatric Psychiatry." **(pp. 530–531)**

Reference

Baltes PB: The aging mind: potential and limits. Gerontologist 33:580–594, 1993